Geriatric Hypertension

Editors

ERIC TUDAY
MARK A. SUPIANO

CLINICS IN GERIATRIC MEDICINE

www.geriatric.theclinics.com

Consulting Editor
G. MICHAEL HARPER

November 2024 • Volume 40 • Number 4

ELSEVIER

1600 John F. Kennedy Boulevard • Suite 1800 • Philadelphia, Pennsylvania, 19103-2899

http://www.theclinics.com

CLINICS IN GERIATRIC MEDICINE Volume 40, Number 4
November 2024 ISSN 0749–0690, ISBN-13: 978-0-443-29694-9

Editor: Taylor Hayes
Developmental Editor: Anita Chamoli

Clinics in Geriatric Medicine (ISSN 0749-0690) is published quarterly by Elsevier Inc., 360 Park Avenue South, New York, NY 10010-1710. Months of issue are February, May, August, and November. Business and Editorial Offices: 1600 John F. Kennedy Blvd., Suite 1800, Philadelphia, PA 191023-2899. Periodicals postage paid at New York, NY, and additional mailing offices. Subscription prices are $321.00 per year (US individuals), $100.00 per year (US & Canadian student/resident), $340.00 per year (Canadian individuals), $457.00 per year (international individuals), and $195.00 per year (international student/resident). For institutional access pricing please contact Customer Service via the contact information below. Foreign air speed delivery is included in all *Clinics* subscription prices. All prices are subject to change without notice. Orders, claims, and journal inquiries: Please visit our Support Hub page https://service.elsevier.com for assistance.

Reprints. For copies of 100 or more, of articles in this publication, please contact the Commercial Reprints Department, Elsevier Inc., 360 Park Avenue South, New York, New York 10010-1710. Tel.: 212-633-3874; Fax: 212-633-3820, E-mail: reprints@elsevier.com.

Clinics in Geriatric Medicine is covered in *MEDLINE/PubMed (Index Medicus), EMBASE/Excerpta Medica, Current Contents/Clinical Medicine (CC/CM),* and the *Cumulative Index to Nursing & Allied Health Literature.*

Contributors

CONSULTING EDITOR

G. MICHAEL HARPER, MD
Professor of Medicine, Geriatrics Department of Medicine, University of California, San Francisco, San Francisco, California, USA

EDITORS

ERIC TUDAY, MD, PhD
Assistant Professor, Division of Cardiovascular Medicine, Department of Internal Medicine, Spencer Eccles Fox School of Medicine, University of Utah, VA Salt Lake City Geriatric Research, Education and Clinical Center, Salt Lake City, Utah, USA

MARK A. SUPIANO, MD, AGSF
Keith Barnes, MD and Dottie Barnes Presidential Endowed Chair in Medicine, Professor, Division of Geriatrics, Professor of Internal Medicine, Spencer Fox Eccles School of Medicine, Executive Director, University of Utah Center on Aging, University of Utah, Salt Lake City, Utah, USA

AUTHORS

WELMA WILDES AMORIM, MD, PhD
Adjunct Professor, Health Sciences Department, State University of Southwest Bahia, Candeias, Brazil

CARTER BAUGHMAN, MD
Resident Physician, Department of Medicine, Beth Israel Deaconess Medical Center, Harvard Medical School, Boston, Massachusetts, USA

ROGER S. BLUMENTHAL, MD
Kenneth Jay Pollin Professor of Cardiology, Director of Johns Hopkins Ciccarone Center for the Prevention of Cardiovascular Disease, Professor of Medicine, Ciccarone Center for the Prevention of Cardiovascular Disease, Johns Hopkins University School of Medicine, Baltimore, Maryland, USA

KENNETH BOOCKVAR, MD, MS
Director, Division of Gerontology, Geriatrics, and Palliative Care, University of Alabama, Birmingham, Alabama, USA

CHRISTOPHER BARRETT BOWLING, MD, MSPH
Associate Professor, Department of Medicine, Duke University, Durham Veterans Affairs Geriatric Research Education and Clinical Center, Durham Veterans Affairs Medical Center (VAMC), Durham, North Carolina, USA

ADAM P. BRESS, PharmD, MS
Associate Professor, Intermountain Healthcare Department of Population Health Sciences, Spencer Fox Eccles School of Medicine, University of Utah, Salt Lake City, Utah, USA

ADAM M. BRICKMAN, PhD
Professor of Neuropsychology, Department of Neurology, Columbia University Medical Center, New York, New York, USA

COLLIN BURKS, MD
Medical Instructor, Department of Medicine, Duke University, Durham, North Carolina, USA

SPENCER V. CARTER, MD
Cardiology Fellow, Division of Cardiology, Department of Internal Medicine, University of Texas Southwestern Medical Center, Dallas, Texas, USA

ALEXANDER CHAITOFF, MD, MPH
Research Fellow, Division of Pharmacoepidemiology and Pharmacoeconomics, Brigham and Women's Hospital, Harvard Medical School, Boston, Massachusetts, USA

ADAM DE HAVENON, MD, MS
Associate Professor, Department of Neurology, Yale University, Center for Brain and Mind Health, Yale University, New Haven, Connecticut, USA

CATHERINE G. DERINGTON, PharmD, MS
Research Assistant Professor, Intermountain Healthcare Department of Population Health Sciences, Spencer Fox Eccles School of Medicine, University of Utah, Salt Lake City, Utah, USA

BRENT M. EGAN, MD
Vice-President, Cardiovascular Health, American Medical Association, Professor of Medicine, Adjunct Professor of Medicine and Nursing, Medical University of South Carolina, Greenville, South Carolina, USA

DEBORAH FURMAN, MD
Resident Physician, Department of Internal Medicine, University of Utah, Salt Lake City, Utah, USA

JOHN M. GIACONA, PhD, PA-C
Assistant Professor, Cardiology Division, Department of Applied Clinical Research, University of Texas Southwestern Medical Center, Dallas, Texas, USA

YUSI GONG, MD
Resident Physician, Department of Medicine, Beth Israel Deaconess Medical Center, Harvard Medical School, Boston, Massachusetts, USA

EMMA HANLON, MD
Resident Physician, Department of Medicine, Beth Israel Deaconess Medical Center, Harvard Medical School, Boston, Massachusetts, USA

CELIA PENA HEREDIA, MD
Physician, Department of Internal Medicine, University of Utah, Salt Lake City, Utah, USA

JOSHUA A. JACOBS, PharmD
Graduate Research Assistant, Intermountain Healthcare Department of Population Health Sciences, Spencer Fox Eccles School of Medicine, University of Utah, Salt Lake City, Utah, USA

STEPHEN JURASCHEK, MD, PhD
Assistant Professor, Department of Medicine, Beth Israel Deaconess Medical Center, Harvard Medical School, Boston, Massachusetts, USA

SVERRE E. KJELDSEN, MD, PhD
Professor Emeritus and Chief Physician, Departments of Cardiology, and Nephrology, Institute of Clinical Medicine, University of Oslo, Senior Consultant, Ullevaal Hospital, Oslo, Norway

MATTHEW KNIGHT, MBBS
Academic Foundation Doctor, Academic Unit for Ageing and Stroke Research, University of Leeds, Leeds, England

LAUREN LITTIG, BA
Clinical Research Associate, Department of Neurology, Yale University, New Haven, Connecticut, USA

EVA A. MISTRY, MBBS, MSCI
Associate Professor, Department of Neurology and Rehabilitation Medicine, University of Cincinnati, Cincinnati, Ohio, USA

PABLO MACIEL MOREIRA, BPharm, MsC
Postgraduate Program in Pharmaceutical Services and Policies, Federal University of Bahia, Salvador, Brazil; Pharmacist, Municipal Health Department of Vitória da Conquista, Vitória da Conquista, Bahia, Brazil

DENISSE G. MORENO, MD
Research Fellow, Division of Geriatrics, Department of Internal Medicine, University of Utah, Salt Lake City, Utah, USA

SHAWNA D. NESBITT, MD, MS
John C. Vanatta III Professor of Medicine, Division of Cardiology, Hypertension Section, Department of Internal Medicine, University of Texas Southwestern Medical Center, Dallas, Texas, USA

MARCIO GALVÃO OLIVEIRA, BPharm, PhD
Associate Professor, Postgraduate Program in Pharmaceutical Services and Policies, Multidisciplinary Institute in Health, Federal University of Bahia, Salvador, Brazil

MICHAEL W. RICH, MD
Professor, Department of Medicine, Washington University School of Medicine, St Louis, Missouri, USA

GARIMA SHARMA, MD
Director of Cardio-Obstetrics and Director of Cardiovascular Women's Health, Inova Schar Heart and Vascular, Inova Health System, Falls Church, Virginia, USA; Ciccarone Center for the Prevention of Cardiovascular Disease, Johns Hopkins University School of Medicine, Baltimore, Maryland, USA

JAMES P. SHEPPARD, PhD
Associate Professor, Nuffield Department of Primary Care Health Sciences, University of Oxford, Oxford, England, United Kingdom

KEVIN N. SHETH, MD
Chief, Neurocritical Care and Emergency Neurology, Department of Neurology, Center for Brain and Mind Health, Yale University, New Haven, Connecticut, USA

DAICHI SHIMBO, MD
Cardiologist and Professor, Department of Medicine, Columbia University Irving Medical Center, New York, New York, USA

JARED A. SPITZ, MD
Physician, Inova Schar Heart and Vascular, Inova Health System, Falls Church, Virginia, USA

MARK A. SUPIANO, MD, AGSF
Keith Barnes, MD and Dottie Barnes Presidential Endowed Chair in Medicine, Professor, Division of Geriatrics, Professor of Internal Medicine, Spencer Fox Eccles School of Medicine, Executive Director, University of Utah Center on Aging, University of Utah, Salt Lake City, Utah, USA

SUSAN E. SUTHERLAND, PhD
Senior Biostatistician, American Medical Association, Greenville, South Carolina, USA

OLIVER M. TODD, MBBS, PhD
Clinical Associate Professor, Academic Unit for Ageing and Stroke Research, University of Leeds, Leeds, England; Bradford Institute for Health Research, Bradford Teaching Hospitals NHS Trust, Bradford, England

ERIC TUDAY, MD, PhD
Assistant Professor, Divisions of Cardiology and Cardiovascular Medicine, Department of Internal Medicine, Spencer Eccles Fox School of Medicine, University of Utah, Physician, Salt Lake City Veterans Affairs Hospital, VA Salt Lake City Geriatric Research, Geriatrics Research Education and Clinical Center (GRECC), Salt Lake City, Utah, USA

WANPEN VONGPATANASIN, MD
Professor of Medicine, Director of the Hypertension Section, Cardiology Division, Department of Internal Medicine, University of Texas Southwestern Medical Center, Dallas, Texas, USA

JACKSON T. WRIGHT JR, MD, PhD
Professor Emeritus, Department of Medicine, College of Medicine, Case Western Reserve University, University Hospitals Case Medical Center, UH Cleveland Medical Center, Cleveland, Ohio, USA

YINGFEI WU, MD, MPH
General Internal Medicine Fellow, Department of Medicine, Massachusetts General Hospital, Harvard Medical School, Boston, Massachusetts, USA

EUGENE YANG, MD, MS
Professor, Division of Cardiology, Department of Medicine, University of Washington School of Medicine, Seattle, Washington, USA; Co-director, Clinical Professor, UW Medicine Cardiovascular Wellness and Prevention Program, Medicine; Chair, Medicine - Eastside Specialty Center, Carl and René e Behnke Endowed Professorship for Asian Health, Bellevue, Washington, USA

ALEXANDER R. ZHEUTLIN, MD, MS
Cardiology Fellow, Division of Cardiology, Feinberg School of Medicine, Northwestern University, Chicago, Illinois, USA

Contents

> The exact definition of hypertension in older adults has changed over the decades, but the benefits of strict blood pressure control across the life span are being increasingly recognized by professional societies and guideline committees. This article discusses the prevalence of hypertension in older adults and describes the associations between hypertension and both clinical and nonclinical morbidity in that population.

> Black and Hispanic older adults in the United States have higher prevalence of hypertension, less adequate treatment, less consistent blood pressure control, and worse cardiovascular outcomes than their white counterparts. Genetic differences are insufficient to explain these disparities—various social, economic, and environmental factors notably contribute. Racial and ethnic differences in living circumstances, household income, access to appropriate care, food security, educational attainment, and tobacco use all negatively impact long-term hypertension outcomes in minoritized older adults. To remedy these inequities, the search for solutions must include a complete assessment of the social, racial, and cultural components of the problem.

> Vascular stiffness is an age-related pathophysiological process that represents a significant risk of cardiovascular morbidity and mortality in the older adult.

> Hypertension impacts most older adults as one of many multiple chronic conditions. A thorough evaluation is required to assess overall health, cardiovascular status, and comorbid conditions that impact treatment targets. In the absence of severe frailty or dementia, intensive treatment prevents more cardiovascular events than standard treatment and may slow cognitive decline. "Start low and go slow" is not the best strategy

CLINICS IN GERIATRIC MEDICINE

ISSUES OF RELATED INTEREST

Medical Clinics
https://www.medical.theclinics.com/
Primary Care: Clinics in Office Practice
https://www.primarycare.theclinics.com/

THE CLINICS ARE AVAILABLE ONLINE!
Access your subscription at:
www.theclinics.com

Foreword

Three Decades of Progress Since the Systolic Hypertension in the Elderly Program

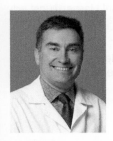

G. Michael Harper, MD
Consulting Editor

I was just beginning my internship when the landmark Systolic Hypertension in the Elderly Program (SHEP) study was published demonstrating the stroke and cardiovascular benefits of treating isolated systolic hypertension (ISH) in adults over the age of 60.[1] The year was 1991, and until that time, there was no consensus that treating ISH in older adults would improve clinical outcomes, and clinicians worried about the safety of treatment, particularly that lowering blood pressure too much or too rapidly could lead to stroke.[2]

Our understanding of high blood pressure, its pathophysiology, measurement methods, treatment, and treatment goals has evolved and advanced over the more than 30 years since the SHEP study and since our last update on hypertension in 2009. In this issue, our guest editors, Drs Mark Supiano and Eric Tuday, have recruited a team of experts who have put together a comprehensive review of hypertension and the special considerations for older adults. The topics covered will enhance our readers' understanding of vascular aging and its role in the development of high blood pressure, the relationship between blood pressure and cognitive function, the non-pharmacologic and pharmacologic treatment of hypertension, and the optimal targets for treatment. Other articles address social, racial, and cultural considerations, long-term monitoring, resistant hypertension, and the potential role of deprescribing.

Just over three decades ago, we were not sure ISH could or should be treated safely. Today, we more fully understand the risks associated with untreated hypertension and how to evaluate and manage it in older adults. I'm confident that readers of this issue

Clin Geriatr Med 40 (2024) xiii–xiv
https://doi.org/10.1016/j.cger.2024.07.002
0749-0690/24/© 2024 Published by Elsevier Inc.

geriatric.theclinics.com

will not only emerge with new knowledge but also have the tools they need to individualize hypertension care for their patients.

G. Michael Harper, MD
Geriatrics Department of Medicine
University of California, San Francisco
4150 Clement Street, Rm 310B
San Francisco, CA 94121, USA

E-mail address:
Michael.Harper@ucsf.edu

REFERENCES

1. Prevention of stroke by antihypertensive drug treatment in older persons with isolated systolic hypertension. Final results of the Systolic Hypertension in the Elderly Program (SHEP). JAMA 1991;265(24):3255–64.
2. Winker MA, Murphy MB. Isolated systolic hypertension in the elderly. JAMA 1991; 265(24):3301–2.

Preface

A Call to Action for Blood Pressure Control in Older Adults

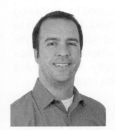 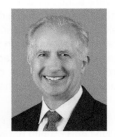

Eric Tuday, MD, PhD   Mark A. Supiano, MD
Editors

High blood pressure (BP) is the leading contributor to preventable death worldwide. The increasing prevalence of elevated BP, the age-associated increase in BP, and the worldwide demographic increase in the aging population are converging to create a serious public health threat. There have been many important updates to the body of evidence available to inform clinicians and patients regarding hypertension in older adults since the last issue of *Clinics in Geriatric Medicine* devoted to Geriatric Hypertension was published in 2009. Perhaps the single most important update is that the threshold now recommended in most clinical guidelines defines hypertension as a systolic BP in excess of 130 mm Hg. This change was driven, in part, by results that have emerged from two randomized clinical trials of intensive BP lowering that have been completed since 2009. In addition to a mortality benefit, additional benefits demonstrable with intensive BP control in older adults were identified in hypertension-related conditions, including cardiovascular and cerebral-vascular events, chronic kidney disease, and cognitive impairment. Indeed, there is now clear evidence that what is good for the heart is good for the brain.

We assembled an international group of experts (from Brazil, England, Mexico, and Norway in addition to faculty from fifteen major US academic medical centers and the American Medical Association) in this topic area to update seven of the 2009 issue's articles: "Epidemiology," "Vascular Aging," "General Principles, Etiologies, Evaluation, and Hypertension Management," "Cognitive Function," "Nonpharmacologic Management," "Pharmacologic Treatment," and "Resistant Hypertension." With one exception, all this issue's authors are new contributors. In addition, this issue has added five new, timely topics: "Social, Racial, and Cultural Considerations," "Long-Term Monitoring: A Focus on Self-Measured Blood Pressure," "Optimal Blood

Clin Geriatr Med 40 (2024) xv–xvi
https://doi.org/10.1016/j.cger.2024.07.001
0749-0690/24/© 2024 Published by Elsevier Inc.

Pressure Targets," "Deprescribing Hypertension Medication," and "Public Health Messaging to Older Adults."

The call to action to improve hypertension awareness and control rates among older adults is even more imperative today. Reducing elevated systolic BP to below 130 mm Hg is one of the few interventions for which there is now clear evidence of benefit to significantly reduce mortality and morbidity, including preventing the development of cognitive impairment in older individuals, inclusive of ambulatory, frail older adults. With the recognition that BP control rates were suboptimal when the threshold was 140 mm Hg, it seems evident that greater attention needs to be devoted to improving systolic BP control rates among the high-risk population of older adults. In addition to implementing the public health messaging strategies outlined in this new article, system level approaches that incorporate geriatric principles (age-friendly care approaches and interprofessional team care) combined with quality improvement strategies urgently need to be adopted to address this public health crisis.

DISCLOSURES

Dr M.A. Supiano reports grant funding from NIH and royalty payments from McGraw-Hill Publishing. Dr E. Tuday reports grant funding from the NIH and Western Institute for Biomedical Research.

Eric Tuday, MD, PhD
Division of Cardiovascular Medicine
Department of Internal Medicine
Spencer Eccles Fox School of Medicine
University of Utah
30 North Mario Capecchi Drive
3rd Floor North
Salt Lake City, UT 84112, USA

Mark A. Supiano, MD
Geriatrics Division
Department of Internal Medicine
University of Utah Center on Aging
University of Utah
30 North Mario Capecchi Drive
2nd Floor North
Salt Lake City, UT 84112, USA

E-mail addresses:
eric.tuday@hsc.utah.edu (E. Tuday)
mark.supiano@utah.edu (M.A. Supiano)

Epidemiology of Hypertension in Older Adults

Alexander Chaitoff, MD, MPH[a],*, Alexander R. Zheutlin, MD, MS[b]

KEYWORDS

• Hypertension • Cardiovascular disease • Older adults • Geriatrics • Epidemiology

KEY POINTS

• There is increasing evidence of benefit to targeting more intensive blood pressure goals in older adults, which are usually defined as ranging from less than 130/80 mm Hg to less than 140/90 mm Hg.
• Less than approximately 10% of adults aged 65 years or older are normotensive without the aid of antihypertensives.
• In adults aged 65 years or older, hypertension has the single largest population attributable fraction of any risk factor for cardiovascular disease.
• A diagnosis of hypertension is associated with multiple psychological and financial consequences.

DEFINING HYPERTENSION AMONG OLDER ADULTS

Describing the epidemiology of hypertension in older adults first requires establishing a common definition of "hypertension" and "older adults."

The definition of "older adult" is not consistent in medical literature. For example, many epidemiologists use the Medicare eligibility age of 65 years or older as the definition of an older adult. In contrast, the Centers for Disease Control includes adults as young as 50 years of age as "older adults" in the scheme of some of their chronic disease indicator definitions.[1] As such, it is unsurprising to see that "older adult" means different people in different studies. Even if a commonly agreed upon age-cutoff existed, older adults are not a homogenous group and prevalence estimates that generalize to the entire group inherently lack nuance. As such, we will first provide age ranges and descriptors of the samples used to obtain the epidemiologic estimates we present.

[a] Division of Pharmacoepidemiology and Pharmacoeconomics, Brigham and Women's Hospital/Harvard Medical School, Boston, MA, USA; [b] Division of Cardiology, Feinberg School of Medicine, Northwestern University, 676 North St. Clair Street, Arkes Suite 2330, Chicago, IL 60611, USA
* Corresponding author. 2014 Washington Street, 3rd Floor, Newton, MA 02462.
E-mail address: amc231@case.edu

Clin Geriatr Med 40 (2024) 515–528
https://doi.org/10.1016/j.cger.2024.04.007
0749-0690/24/© 2024 Elsevier Inc. All rights reserved.
geriatric.theclinics.com

As for hypertension, the definition has evolved over the years as has our understanding of when to treat hypertension in older adults. Understanding this context is important as not all time periods had clinically agreed upon definitions of hypertension and thus can skew epidemiologic estimates.

Historical Context of Hypertension in Older Adults

In the early twentieth century, contemporary medical opinion was to not treat asymptomatic patients with blood pressures up to (and even over) 180/110 mm Hg regardless of age.[2] There were several reasons physicians were hesitant to treat patients. Notably, there was limited evidence for the dangers of essential hypertension, which was regularly referred to as "benign" essential hypertension. Moreover, treatments for high blood pressure were scarcely available and often poorly tolerated.[3] This combination of the perceived benign nature of hypertension and limited treatment options led the medical community away from classifying hypertension as a serious health risk that required intervention.

However, innovation and evidence generated from the late 1950s through 1970 set the stage for the National High Blood Pressure Education Program and subsequently the first widely circulated guidelines for treating hypertension. Specifically, new, well-tolerated oral medications (notably the thiazide class of diuretics) came to the market and 2 pivotal trials proved that treating hypertension improved clinical outcomes.[4-6] This evidence informed Joint National Committee (JNC) I, the first national recommendations for treating patients with diastolic blood pressures greater than 90 mm Hg.[7]

Despite evidence in the 1970s suggesting systolic, versus diastolic, blood pressure more closely associated with coronary heart disease, it was not until JNC V (1992) that the importance of a systolic blood pressure (SBP) goal was codified by guideline recommendations.[8-10] Through JNC VII (2003), goal blood pressures for older adults (defined as >60 or >65 years of age in different recommendations) generally mirrored those for younger adults.[11] Though not a formal guideline, in 2014, the authors of JNC VIII published their recommendations that broke from prior and contemporary guidelines at the time by recommending not initiating pharmacologic treatment in adults aged older than 60 years if their blood pressure was less than 150/90 mm Hg.[12] This was based largely on 2 null trials, one of which may have been underpowered and included relatively healthy older adults and one that did have a significant interaction between age and development of cardiovascular or renal disease.[13,14] Though JNC VIII was published as a single recommendation, the authors note in the recommendation itself that there were disagreements about this topic on the panel.

Current Recommendations

The current era in hypertension management of older adults is primarily informed by 2 pivotal trials. The Hypertension in the Very Elderly Trial (HYVET), published in 2008, suggested it was beneficial to treat older adults with particularly poor hypertension control (HYVET, for example, included adults aged 80 years or older with SBPs >160 mm Hg).[15] However, the most influential data informing more recent guidelines' stringent hypertension definitions are from the Systolic Blood Pressure Intervention Trial (SPRINT) published in 2015.[16] In this trial, 9361 patients with SBP greater than 130 mm Hg and an increased cardiovascular risk (but not diabetes) were randomized to an intensive (SBP <120 mm Hg) or standard (SBP <140 mm Hg) blood pressure target and followed for a median 3.26 years to assess for cardiovascular events and death. The trial found that those randomized to the intensive target had a 25% and 27% reduction in the hazard of cardiovascular events and all-cause mortality, respectively. A subgroup analysis limited to the 2636 patients who were aged 75 years or older as well as meta-analyses of multiple trials have subsequently been published showing similar results.[17,18] While these 2 trials have had the largest influence on guidelines in the United States, there are others, notably the STEP trial performed in China, confirming the benefits of intensive blood pressure control even in older adults.[19]

Since 2017, these data have led professional societies to recognize the benefits of more intensive blood pressure targets, which usually range from less than 130/80 mm Hg to less than 140/90 mm Hg. Of note, though evidence continues to be generated on the topics, current guidelines only sparsely comment on isolated diastolic hypertension or J-curve phenomena in older adults, which could be in part due to less clear evidence about how this translates to cardiovascular disease risk in this population.[20–22]

Given this history, defining hypertension in older adults is somewhat era-specific. To be consistent with the last 20 years of clinical recommendations, quality measures (eg, Healthcare Effectiveness Data and Information Set measures), and epidemiologic practices, we generally use the threshold of 140/90 mm Hg for the purposes of defining hypertension throughout the remainder of this report despite evidence that more intensive control (ie, <130/80 mm Hg) may have additional cardiovascular benefit.

HYPERTENSION IN OLDER ADULTS

Over the life span, there is cumulative exposure to endothelial damaging events, increasing the risk of arterial stiffness, impaired vascular reactivity, and hemodynamic shifts that can further propagate arterial dysfunction.[23–26] As the likelihood of vascular dysfunction increases with age, the ability to maintain normal blood pressure and variability decreases over time. This change leads to a lower prevalence of ideal blood pressure in older adults with a phenotypic pattern that classically includes a wide pulse pressure with SBP elevations that are relatively greater than diastolic blood pressure elevations.[26] Data from National Health and Nutrition Examination Survey (NHANES) demonstrated that between 2011 and 2018, only 11.2% and 5% of adults aged 65 to 74 years and 75 years or older had a blood pressure of less than 120/80 mm Hg.[27]

Epidemiology of Hypertension in Older Adults

Among adults in the United States, the prevalence of hypertension increases with age. Through much of the twenty-first century, the prevalence of hypertension in older adults has remained relatively consistent (**Fig. 1**). From 2009 and 2012, the prevalence of hypertension (blood pressure >140/90 mm Hg) was 63.9% and 76.8% among adults aged 65 to 74 years and 75 years or older, respectively.[28] From 2017 through 2020, the prevalence among adults aged 65 to 74 years and 75 years or older was 64.1% and 74.5%, respectively.[28] However, hypertension awareness has fallen among older adults: from 2012 through 2017, fewer adults aged 75 years or older were aware they were hypertensive compared to adults examined between 2009 through 2012 (79.6% vs 86.0%; $P = .019$).[28]

Despite a greater prevalence of hypertension among older adults compared to younger adults, underdiagnosis remains a common problem faced by older adults and may impact awareness of disease. Among adults without elevated clinic blood pressure, it is estimated that the prevalence of masked hypertension is 28.0% in adults aged 65 years or older.[29] Diurnal variation in blood pressure may differentially impact older adults as well. Based on a threshold of greater than 140/90 mm Hg, an estimated 27.2% of adults aged 65 years or older have masked hypertension while asleep only, leaving them vulnerable to a missed diagnosis of hypertension.[30]

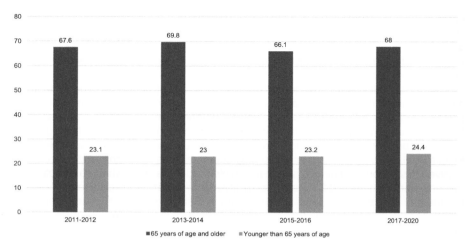

Fig. 1. Prevalence of hypertension among adults aged 65 years or older versus younger than 65 years within the United States. Hypertension is defined as a blood pressure greater than 140/90 mm Hg or self-reported antihypertensive medication use. (Data are available via the Centers for Disease Control and Prevention National Health Examination and Nutrition Survey 2011–2020.)

It is important to note that many estimates of hypertension, including the preceding prevalences, come from national surveys that do not sample institutionalized adults. Selection bias is a concern in all survey research, but survey estimates are at particularly high risk of mischaracterizing certain older adults if they exclude homebound or nursing home residents. Hypertension is common among older adults living in nursing homes. Though estimates vary, studies consistently find at least 50% of nursing home residents have measured blood pressure greater than 140/90 mm Hg and greater than 75% are on antihypertensive medications.[31–33]

Beyond overall estimates, there are key disparities in hypertension prevalence within the United States among older adults. Hypertension is nearly 5 percentage points more prevalent among women aged 65 years or older than among men in the same age range (70.2% vs 65.4%; threshold of >140/90 mm Hg), which is despite similar awareness rates (women: 60.4% vs men: 57.6%).[34] Interestingly, this prevalence gap does narrow when using a threshold of greater than 130/80 mm Hg (women 78.2% vs men: 76.4%).[34]

Differences in hypertension prevalence among older adults also exist by race and ethnicity. Whereas older (≥65 year) non-Hispanic White adults have a hypertension prevalence of 64.5%, non-Hispanic Black, non-Hispanic Asian, and Hispanic adults have prevalences of 87.4%, 79.6%, and 73.8%, respectively. This contrasts with a lower prevalence of hypertension awareness among older non-Hispanic White adults (56.3%), compared to non-Hispanic Black, non-Hispanic Asian, and Hispanic adults (78.2%, 61.4%, and 62.3%, respectively).[34]

Further, the predisposition to develop hypertension appears to be greater among older adults without a high school degree as well as those with low income and accumulated wealth.[35] Just as individual-level socioeconomic factors are being associated with incident hypertension among older adults, so too are neighborhood-level socioeconomic factors. Older adults living in neighborhoods with a lower average socioeconomic status have higher incident hypertension than those living in the neighborhoods with the highest socioeconomic status.[36] Despite increased efforts to reduce the burden of hypertension among older adults, the prevalence of hypertension has remained stable over the past decade with sparse improvements in disparities faced by minoritized older adults with hypertension (**Fig. 2**).

Blood pressure control among older adults with hypertension remains a challenge. Though the prevalence of older adults who are both aware they have hypertension and are taking an antihypertensive medication is over 95%, only 36.8% of adults aged 75 years or older have a blood pressure less than 140/90 mm Hg overall, and only 47.7% among those are taking an antihypertensive medication.[27] Even with a multi-agent strategy to treat hypertension among older adults, blood pressure control can be difficult to achieve, and pooled analysis of participants from the NHANES between 2009 and 2014 found that 47.8% of adults aged 70 years or older met criteria for apparent treatment-resistant hypertension.[37] Some of this may be due to inadequate uptitration of antihypertensive regimens: for example, only 12.5% of adults aged 60 years or older with hypertension were appropriately intensified on antihypertensive therapy during clinic visits between 2015 and 2018.[38]

Frailty and fear of causing older adults harm is often cited as a reason for insufficient blood pressure management for older adults; however, clinical inertia is prevalent among older adults regardless of cognitive or physical function status.[39,40] Furthermore, post hoc analyses of HYVET and SPRINT demonstrate that frail adults derive significant benefit from appropriate blood pressure control.[41,42] Moreover, in a subgroup analysis of adults aged 75 years or older from SPRINT, the prevalence of serious adverse events was higher among older adults compared with their younger counterparts but was not actually not different between older adults randomized to an intensive versus standard blood pressure target.[17] As such, frailty and fear of adverse drug events should perhaps have less influence on the epidemiology of antihypertensive use and disease control than it does in the current landscape.

Hypertension is highly prevalent, especially in certain groups, and remains poorly controlled in many older adults. Though elevated blood pressure leads to significant morbidity and mortality, proper diagnosis and treatment of older adults with hypertension remain a key challenge facing a growing aging population.

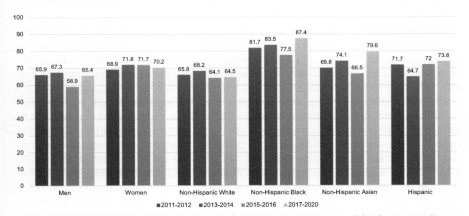

Fig. 2. Prevalence of hypertension among adults aged 65 years or older by sex and race/ethnicity within the United States between 2011 and 2020. Hypertension is defined as a blood pressure greater than 140/90 mm Hg or self-reported antihypertensive medication use. (Data are available via the Centers for Disease Control and Prevention National Health Examination and Nutrition Survey 2011–2020.)

CLINICAL MANIFESTATIONS OF HYPERTENSION IN OLDER ADULTS

Hypertension itself rarely causes symptoms, though it is the leading modifiable risk factor of disease involving multiple organ systems including the heart, brain, and kidneys.[43,44] Most notably, hypertension is arguably the most prevalent and penetrant risk factor for cardiovascular disease in older adults: one study estimated that, in adults aged greater than 60 years, the population attributable fraction of hypertension for cardiovascular disease was 14.1% (95% confidence interval [CI] 12.7%–15.5%), the highest percentage for any single risk factor.[45]

It is well publicized that cardiovascular disease is the foremost cause of death in the United States.[46] However, this is actually only true for older adults. Among adults aged 65 years or older, over 525,000 deaths are attributable to cardiovascular disease each year.[47] Given the primary purpose of diagnosing and treating hypertension is often to reduce the risk of cardiovascular disease, understanding its impact in older adults is paramount.

Epidemiology of Cardiovascular Disease in Older Adults

Much like describing the scope of hypertension in older adults, doing the same for cardiovascular disease is a complicated task for several reasons. First, cardiovascular disease is a broad term. For example, when identifying cause of death, ischemic heart disease is classified as cardiovascular disease while strokes are often classified separately as "cerebrovascular disease," but in other clinical studies, strokes are often included as cardiovascular events. The variability of conditions that fit under the umbrella term of cardiovascular disease obscures efforts to understand the true burden of disease. This is in addition to the challenges described earlier, which include the issue of treating older adults as a homogenous group and the fact that the definition of "older adult" varies in the literature.

Regardless of which specific diseases and which specific age ranges are included, cardiovascular disease is common among older adults (**Fig. 3**). Among all adults, the prevalence of heart disease (defined in this case as coronary artery disease, heart failure, or stroke) is 9.9%; however, the prevalence is more than double that among adults aged 65 years or older.[48] Notably, those with hypertension are more likely to have all forms of heart disease (**Fig. 4**).

Concerning incidence, one large study of pooled data of several US-based prospective cohorts (n = 19,630) assessed rates of new cardiovascular disease among adults aged 55 to 85 years. In 272,124 person-years of follow-up, the incidental proportion of cardiovascular disease (defined more narrowly as including only coronary artery disease or stroke) ranged from 15.3% to 38.6% for women and from 21.5% to 47.7% for men, which depended on other baseline cardiometabolic risk factors.[49]

Aside from traditional cardiometabolic risk factors, it is as important to recognize the relationships between various socioeconomic and demographic factors with cardiovascular disease in older adults. Notably, there are higher rates of cardiovascular mortality in both Black women (rate ratio [RR] 1.32, 95% CI 1.30–1.33) and Black men (RR 1.33, 95% CI 1.32–1.34) compared with their White counterparts, though the differences in cardiovascular mortality rates are smaller in magnitude among older adults than they are among patients aged less than 65 years.[50] There are several hypotheses for why there is a slight narrowing of disparities after 65 years, but the impact of insurance coverage (ie, qualifying for Medicare) is one that has been proven empirically.[51] Still, Medicare is not a cure-all, and significant disparities in cardiovascular disease morbidity remain among older adults across several socioeconomic axes.[52,53] For example, in a sample of 128,789 Medicare beneficiaries prior strokes, Black patients

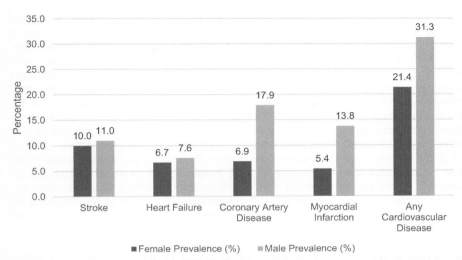

Fig. 3. Prevalence of self-reported cardiovascular disease among adults aged 65 years or older stratified by sex. (Data are available via the Centers for Disease Control and Prevention National Health Examination and Nutrition Survey 2017–2020.)

(compared with White ones) were significantly more likely to have recurrent strokes within 1 year (hazard ratio [HR] 1.36, 95% CI 1.29–1.44).[54]

As dependence on others may increase as adults age, social support and living situations play significant roles in the socioeconomic considerations associated with cardiovascular disease in older adults. Neighborhood deprivation has been

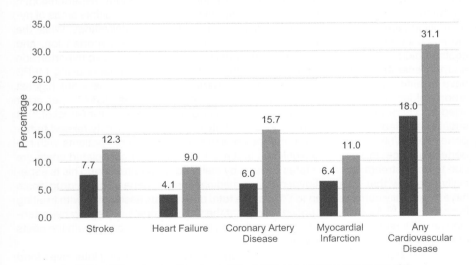

Fig. 4. Prevalence of self-reported cardiovascular disease among adults aged 65 years or older stratified by self-reported hypertensive status. (Data are available via the Centers for Disease Control and Prevention National Health Examination and Nutrition Survey 2017–202.)

shown to be a particularly strong correlate with cardiovascular disease risk in older adults. In a study longitudinally following 288,555 participants aged 51 to 70 years enrolled in the National Institutes of Health-AARP (NIH-AARP) Diet and Health Study, increases in neighborhood deprivation over time were associated with greater cardiovascular mortality. Participants living in neighborhoods that became increasingly deprived over time faced significantly greater risk of cardiovascular mortality compared with those who started in and remained in the neighborhoods with the least deprivation (HR 1.76, 95% CI 1.41–2.19).[55] Feelings of isolation have similarly been associated with cardiovascular disease, which is concerning given over 33% of adults aged 50 to 80 years report feeling isolated.[56] In one prospective study of 57,825 community-dwelling women (mean age 79 years), high reported social isolation (vs low) was associated with an 18% increased risk of major cardiovascular events.[57] There are many potential mechanisms through which the association between socioeconomic factors and cardiovascular disease may be mediated by increased blood pressure, which could include the stress response or the impact of issues like hypertension treatment adherence.[58,59]

NONCLINICAL IMPACTS OF HYPERTENSION IN OLDER ADULTS

Hypertension impacts patients beyond the clinical manifestations of the downstream diseases it causes. Hypertension and its sequelae can lead to financial toxicity and lost "productivity" time, furthering its deleterious impact in older adults.

Financial Costs Associated with Hypertension

Overall, data from the 2003 to 2014 Medical Expenditure Panel Survey (MEPS) show that patients with hypertension have unadjusted mean health care expenditures of greater than US$9000 per year, which is more than US$1900 per year higher than unadjusted mean health care expenditures of individuals without hypertension.[60] Furthermore, these increased health care costs were seen across multiple areas of hypertension care, from spending on medication to inpatient hospitalizations. While the aforementioned study did not test the interaction between age, hypertension, and costs, it did show that as adults age, they are both more likely to have hypertension and to generate relatively higher health care costs.[60] Other estimates using MEPS have stratified by age and demonstrated hypertension-specific costs are highest among older adults. In 2010, the yearly mean expenditure was US$778 per adult aged 65 years or older with approximately 20% of costs being out-of-pocket.[61] It should be noted this latter estimate includes only costs of care directly related to hypertension. When compared with the total health care expenditures patients with hypertension face, this estimate highlights that most hypertension-associated costs are due to downstream disease-states caused by elevated blood pressure. This is especially true now that most antihypertensive medications are generic given drug costs have historically comprised up to 80% of the total direct costs associated with treating hypertension.[62] As such, it is unsurprising that the financial costs of treating hypertension are now relatively low and in fact continuing to decrease compared with the costs of complications from hypertension.[63]

From a system and value standpoint, evidence suggests that having intensive blood pressure targets for older adults is cost-effective at the population level (US$25,417 per quality-adjusted life year). This would make treating hypertension cost-effective even using relatively strict thresholds from the Institute for Clinical Effectiveness Research and accounting for costs associated with clinic visits and laboratory monitoring, drug costs, and costs of treating adverse events.[64]

Burdens Associated with Carrying a Diagnosis of Hypertension

The diagnosis of hypertension has long been described as coming with a "labeling effect" or a psychological anguish of being diagnosed with the disease that can impair quality of life.[65] One study, which was not limited to older adults (mean age 51.7 years), compared psychological distress in patients who had been labeled as having hypertension versus patients with hypertension but without a diagnosis versus normotensive patients. The authors found higher risk of distress in patients with a hypertension diagnosis, but not those with undiagnosed hypertension, even when adjusted for other health factors.[66]

Medications can also have a profound impact on quality of life. For example, in one survey of Medicare patients, the majority indicated that they would prefer to take fewer medications.[67] Moreover, in cohorts of older adults, polypharmacy and medication appropriateness are correlated with quality of life scores.[68,69] Patients with hypertension, which usually requires 2 or more medications in order to obtain optimal control, are at an increased risk of suffering from polypharmacy, which is also correlated with lower likelihood of achieving blood pressure goals.[70] Fixed-dose combination antihypertensive medication could help alleviate this burden, but appropriate use is less likely among adults aged greater than 60 years compared to adults aged less than 40 years (odds ratio 0.56 95% CI, 0.37–0.83).[71]

Of course, while important to consider, this is not an argument against diagnosing or treating patients with hypertension; rather, it speaks to the importance of confirming diagnoses, careful counseling, and appropriate treatment. Interestingly, among adults with hypertension, there is evidence that patients with well-controlled blood pressure actually have better quality of life than their peers with blood pressures not at goal, which has been shown to be true even in older adults.[72–74] Moreover, estimates extrapolated from the Optimising Treatment for Mild Systolic Hypertension in the Elderly trial suggest it is not cost-effective to deprescribe antihypertensive medications in many older adults, and other research suggests deprescribing interventions more generally have not been shown to improve clinical events or reduce health care utilization.[75,76]

SUMMARY

Hypertension is more prevalent and associated with more morbidity in older adults than it is in any other age group. As such, it is paramount to accurately diagnose hypertension and use shared decision-making approaches to initiate and titrate effective antihypertensive treatment, which can help prevent multiple diseases and ensure value-concordant care.

CLINICS CARE POINTS

- There are cardiovascular benefits to achieving blood pressure control (<140/90 mm Hg) in older adults, and there may be additional benefits to achieving strict control (<130/80 mm Hg).
- Hypertension is highly prevalent in older adults, and all older adults should be screened for hypertension regardless of frailty.
- Hypertension is arguably the number one contributor to heart disease in older adults, and antihypertensive treatment should be considered for all older adults regardless of frailty.

DISCLOSURE

The authors have nothing to disclose.

REFERENCES

1. Centers for Disease Control and Provention. Indicator definitions - older adults. 2015. Available at: https://www.cdc.gov/cdi/definitions/older-adults.html#OLD3_2.
2. Evans W. Hypertension. In: Hoeber Paul B, editor. Cardiology. London: Butterworths Medical Publishing; 1948. p. 204.
3. Moser M. Historical perspectives on the management of hypertension. J Clin Hypertens 2006;8:15–20.
4. Moser M, Macaulay AI. Chlorothiazide as an adjunct in the treatment of essential hypertension. Am J Cardiol 1959;3(2):214–9.
5. Veterans Administration Cooperative Study Group on Antihypertensive Agents. Effects of treatment on morbidity in hypertension. Results in patients with diastolic blood pressures averaging 115 through 129mmHg. JAMA 1967;202:1028–34.
6. Veterans Administration Cooperative Study Group on Antihypertensive Agents. Effects of treatment on morbidity in hypertension, II: results in patients with diastolic pressure averaging 90 through 114 mmHg. JAMA 1970;213(7):1143–52.
7. Committee JN. Report of the Joint National Committee on detection, evaluation, and treatment of high blood pressure. A cooperative study. JAMA 1977;237(3): 255–61.
8. Kannel WB, Gordon T, Schwartz MJ. Systolic versus diastolic blood pressure and risk of coronary heart disease: the Framingham study. Am J Cardiol 1971;27(4): 335–46.
9. Kotchen TA. Developing hypertension guidelines: an evolving process. Am J Hypertens 2014;27(6):765–72.
10. Dustan HP. 50th anniversary historical article. Hypertension. J Am Coll Cardiol 1999;33(3):595–7.
11. Chobanian AV, Bakris GL, Black HR, et al. The seventh report of the joint national committee on prevention, detection, evaluation, and treatment of high blood pressure: the JNC 7 report. JAMA 2003;289(19):2560–71.
12. James PA, Oparil S, Carter BL, et al. 2014 evidence-based guideline for the management of high blood pressure in adults: report from the panel members appointed to the Eighth Joint National Committee (JNC 8). JAMA 2014;311(5): 507–20.
13. JATOS Study Group. Principal results of the Japanese trial to assess optimal systolic blood pressure in elderly hypertensive patients (JATOS). Hypertens Res 2008;31(12):2115–27.
14. Ogihara T, Saruta T, Rakugi H, et al. Target blood pressure for treatment of isolated systolic hypertension in the elderly: valsartan in elderly isolated systolic hypertension study. Hypertension 2010;56(2):196–202.
15. Beckett NS, Peters R, Fletcher AE, et al. Treatment of hypertension in patients 80 years of age or older. N Engl J Med 2008;358(18):1887–98.
16. Group SR. A randomized trial of intensive versus standard blood-pressure control. N Engl J Med 2015;373(22):2103–16.
17. Williamson JD, Supiano MA, Applegate WB, et al. Intensive vs standard blood pressure control and cardiovascular disease outcomes in adults aged$\geq$ 75 years: a randomized clinical trial. JAMA 2016;315(24):2673–82.

18. Rahimi K, Bidel Z, Nazarzadeh M, et al. Age-stratified and blood-pressure-stratified effects of blood-pressure-lowering pharmacotherapy for the prevention of cardiovascular disease and death: an individual participant-level data meta-analysis. Lancet 2021;398(10305):1053–64.
19. Zhang W, Zhang S, Deng Y, et al. Trial of intensive blood-pressure control in older patients with hypertension. N Engl J Med 2021;385(14):1268–79.
20. Filippone EJ, Foy AJ, Naccarelli GV. The diastolic blood pressure J-curve revisited: an update. Am Hear J Plus Cardiol Res Pract 2021;12:100065.
21. Benetos A, Petrovic M, Strandberg T. Hypertension Management in Older and Frail Older Patients. Circ Res 2019;124(7):1045–60.
22. Li J, Somers VK, Gao X, et al. Evaluation of optimal diastolic blood pressure range among adults with treated systolic blood pressure less than 130 mm Hg. JAMA Netw Open 2021;4(2):e2037554.
23. Fonck E, Feigl GG, Fasel J, et al. Effect of aging on elastin functionality in human cerebral arteries. Stroke 2009;40(7):2552–6.
24. AlGhatrif M, Strait JB, Morrell CH, et al. Longitudinal trajectories of arterial stiffness and the role of blood pressure: the Baltimore Longitudinal Study of Aging. Hypertension 2013;62(5):934–41.
25. Safar ME, Thomas F, Blacher J, et al. Metabolic syndrome and age-related progression of aortic stiffness. J Am Coll Cardiol 2006;47(1):72–5.
26. Oliveros E, Patel H, Kyung S, et al. Hypertension in older adults: assessment, management, and challenges. Clin Cardiol 2020;43(2):99–107.
27. Muntner P, Jaeger BC, Hardy ST, et al. Age-specific prevalence and factors associated with normal blood pressure among US adults. Am J Hypertens 2022;35(4):319–27.
28. Muntner P, Miles MA, Jaeger BC, et al. Blood pressure control among US adults, 2009 to 2012 through 2017 to 2020. Hypertension 2022;79(9):1971–80.
29. Wang YC, Shimbo D, Muntner P, et al. Prevalence of masked hypertension among US adults with nonelevated clinic blood pressure. Am J Epidemiol 2017;185(3):194–202.
30. Li S, Schwartz JE, Shimbo D, et al. Estimated prevalence of masked asleep hypertension in US adults. JAMA Cardiol 2021;6(5):568–73.
31. Simonson W, Han LF, Davidson HE. Hypertension treatment and outcomes in US nursing homes: results from the US National Nursing Home Survey. J Am Med Dir Assoc 2011;12(1):44–9.
32. Moore KL, Boscardin WJ, Steinman MA, et al. Age and sex variation in prevalence of chronic medical conditions in older residents of us. nursing homes. J Am Geriatr Soc 2012;60(4):756–64.
33. Liu X, Steinman MA, Lee SJ, et al. Systolic blood pressure, antihypertensive treatment, and cardiovascular and mortality risk in VA nursing home residents. J Am Geriatr Soc 2023;71(7):2131–40.
34. Jaeger BC, Chen L, Foti K, et al. Hypertension statistics for US Adults: an open-source web application for analysis and visualization of national health and nutrition examination survey data. Hypertension 2023;80(6):1311–20.
35. Neufcourt L, Zins M, Berkman LF, et al. Socioeconomic disparities and risk of hypertension among older Americans: the Health and Retirement Study. J Hypertens 2021;39(12):2497–505.
36. McDoom MM, Palta P, Vart P, et al. Late life socioeconomic status and hypertension in an aging cohort: the Atherosclerosis Risk in Communities Study. J Hypertens 2018;36(6):1382.

37. Carey RM, Sakhuja S, Calhoun DA, et al. Prevalence of apparent treatment-resistant hypertension in the United States: comparison of the 2008 and 2018 American Heart Association scientific statements on resistant hypertension. Hypertension 2019;73(2):424–31.

38. Chiu N, Chiu L, Aggarwal R, et al. Trends in blood pressure treatment intensification in older adults with hypertension in the United States, 2008 to 2018. Hypertension 2023;80(3):553–62.

39. Zheutlin AR, Addo DK, Jacobs JA, et al. Evidence for age bias contributing to therapeutic inertia in blood pressure management: a secondary analysis of SPRINT. Hypertension 2023;80(7):1484–93.

40. Hiura GT, Markossian TW, Probst BD, et al. Age and comorbidities are associated with therapeutic inertia among older adults with uncontrolled blood pressure. Am J Hypertens 2024;37(4):280–9.

41. Wang Z, Du X, Hua C, et al. The effect of frailty on the efficacy and safety of intensive blood pressure control: a post hoc analysis of the SPRINT trial. Circulation 2023;148(7):565–74.

42. Warwick J, Falaschetti E, Rockwood K, et al. No evidence that frailty modifies the positive impact of antihypertensive treatment in very elderly people: an investigation of the impact of frailty upon treatment effect in the HYpertension in the Very Elderly Trial (HYVET) study, a double-blind, placeb. BMC Med 2015;13(1):1–8.

43. Burnier M, Damianaki A. Hypertension as cardiovascular risk factor in chronic kidney disease. Circ Res 2023;132(8):1050–63.

44. Reitz C, Tang M-X, Manly J, et al. Hypertension and the risk of mild cognitive impairment. Arch Neurol 2007;64(12):1734–40.

45. Tian F, Chen L, Qian ZM, et al. Ranking age-specific modifiable risk factors for cardiovascular disease and mortality: evidence from a population-based longitudinal study. EClinicalMedicine 2023;64.

46. Ahmad FB, Anderson RN. The leading causes of death in the US for 2020. JAMA 2021;325(18):1829–30.

47. Centers for Disease Control and Provention. Mortality statistics. 2018. Available at: https://www.cdc.gov/injury/wisqars/pdf/leading_causes_of_death_by_age_group_2018-508.pdf.

48. Tsao CW, Aday AW, Almarzooq ZI, et al. Heart disease and stroke statistics—2023 update: a report from the American Heart Association. Circulation 2023;147(8):e93–621.

49. Bancks MP, Ning H, Allen NB, et al. Long-term absolute risk for cardiovascular disease stratified by fasting glucose level. Diabetes Care 2019;42(3):457–65.

50. Kyalwazi AN, Loccoh EC, Brewer LC, et al. Disparities in cardiovascular mortality between Black and White adults in the United States, 1999 to 2019. Circulation 2022;146(3):211–28.

51. McWilliams JM, Meara E, Zaslavsky AM, et al. Differences in control of cardiovascular disease and diabetes by race, ethnicity, and education: US trends from 1999 to 2006 and effects of medicare coverage. Ann Intern Med 2009;150(8):505–15.

52. Faselis C, Safren L, Allman RM, et al. Income disparity and incident cardiovascular disease in older Americans. Prog Cardiovasc Dis 2022;71:92–9.

53. Loccoh EC, Joynt Maddox KE, Wang Y, et al. Rural-urban disparities in outcomes of myocardial infarction, heart failure, and stroke in the United States. J Am Coll Cardiol 2022;79(3):267–79.

54. Albright KC, Huang L, Blackburn J, et al. Racial differences in recurrent ischemic stroke risk and recurrent stroke case fatality. Neurology 2018;91(19):e1741–50.

55. Xiao Q, Berrigan D, Powell-Wiley TM, et al. Ten-year change in neighborhood socioeconomic deprivation and rates of total, cardiovascular disease, and cancer mortality in older US adults. Am J Epidemiol 2018;187(12):2642–50.

56. National Poll on Healthy Aging. Trends in loneliness among older adults from 2018–2023. Available at: https://deepblue.lib.umich.edu/bitstream/handle/2027.42/175971/0300_NPHA-Loneliness-report-FINAL-doifinal.pdf?sequence=4&isAllowed=y.

57. Golaszewski NM, LaCroix AZ, Godino JG, et al. Evaluation of social isolation, loneliness, and cardiovascular disease among older women in the US. JAMA Netw Open 2022;5(2):e2146461.

58. Forde AT, Sims M, Muntner P, et al. Discrimination and hypertension risk among african Americans in the jackson heart study. Hypertension 2020;76(3):715–23.

59. Lu J, Zhang N, Mao D, et al. How social isolation and loneliness effect medication adherence among elderly with chronic diseases: an integrated theory and validated cross-sectional study. Arch Gerontol Geriatr 2020;90:104154.

60. Kirkland EB, Heincelman M, Bishu KG, et al. Trends in healthcare expenditures among US adults with hypertension: national estimates, 2003–2014. J Am Heart Assoc 2018;7(11):e008731.

61. Davis K. Expenditures for hypertension among adults age 18 and older, 2010: estimates for the US civilian noninstitutionalized population. Statistical brief No 404. April 2013. Rockville: Agency for Healthcare Research and Quality; 2014.

62. Odell TW, Gregory MC. Cost of hypertension treatment. J Gen Intern Med 1995; 10(12):686–8.

63. Johansen ME, Byrd JB. Total and out-of-pocket expenditures on antihypertensive medications in the United States, 2007–2019. Hypertension 2021;78(5):1662–4.

64. Liao C-T, Toh HS, Sun L, et al. Cost-effectiveness of intensive vs standard blood pressure control among older patients with hypertension. JAMA Netw Open 2023;6(2):e230708.

65. Wenger NK. Quality of life issues in hypertension: consequences of diagnosis and considerations in management. Am Heart J 1988;116(2):628–32.

66. Hamer M, Batty GD, Stamatakis E, et al. Hypertension awareness and psychological distress. Hypertension 2010;56(3):547–50.

67. Reeve E, Wolff JL, Skehan M, et al. Assessment of attitudes toward deprescribing in older Medicare beneficiaries in the United States. JAMA Intern Med 2018; 178(12):1673–80.

68. Aljeaidi MS, Haaksma ML, Tan ECK. Polypharmacy and trajectories of health-related quality of life in older adults: an Australian cohort study. Qual Life Res 2022;31(9):2663–71.

69. Nordin Olsson I, Runnamo R, Engfeldt P. Medication quality and quality of life in the elderly, a cohort study. Health Qual Life Outcomes 2011;9(1):1–9.

70. Derington CG, Gums TH, Bress AP, et al. Association of total medication burden with intensive and standard blood pressure control and clinical outcomes: a secondary analysis of SPRINT. Hypertension 2019;74(2):267–75.

71. Mobley CM, Bryan AS, Moran AE, et al. Fixed-dose combination medication use among US adults with hypertension: a missed opportunity. J Am Heart Assoc 2023;12(4):e027486.

72. Applegate WB, Pressel S, Wittes J, et al. Impact of the treatment of isolated systolic hypertension on behavioral variables: results from the systolic hypertension in the elderly program. Arch Intern Med 1994;154(19):2154–60.

73. Wiklund I, Halling K, Rydén-Bergsten T, et al. Does lowering the blood pressure improve the mood? quality-of-life results from the hypertension optimal treatment (HOT) study. Blood Press 1997;6(6):357–64.

74. Grimm RH, Grandits GA, Cutler JA, et al. Relationships of quality-of-life measures to long-term lifestyle and drug treatment in the treatment of mild hypertension study. Arch Intern Med 1997;157(6):638–48.

75. Jowett S, Kodabuckus S, Ford GA, et al. Cost-effectiveness of antihypertensive deprescribing in primary care: a Markov modelling study using data from the OPTiMISE trial. Hypertension 2022;79(5):1122–31.

76. Keller MS, Qureshi N, Mays AM, et al. Cumulative update of a systematic overview evaluating interventions addressing polypharmacy. JAMA Netw Open 2024;7(1):e2350963.

Social, Racial, and Cultural Considerations in Hypertension in Older Adults

Shawna D. Nesbitt, MD, MS[a],*, Spencer V. Carter, MD[b]

KEYWORDS

- Hypertension • Disparities • Health equity • Older persons • Race • Ethnicity
- Culture • Social determinants of health

KEY POINTS

- Health disparities exist in hypertension in older persons.
- Disparities in hypertensive older persons are linked to social, cultural, and racial and ethnic differences in the social determinants of health.
- Reducing inequity in hypertension in older persons requires a complex approach that includes commitment from physicians, health care systems, and governmental and community organizations.

INTRODUCTION

Older persons who are African Americans/black and Hispanic have nearly 3 times the rate of disability due to hypertension compared to whites. Physiologic differences by race and ethnicity are insufficient to explain this degree of disparity in hypertension outcomes. This article will examine the problem of hypertension disparities in older persons, contributing factors, and solutions to consider.

THE PROBLEM

Elevated blood pressure contributes heavily to excess morbidity and mortality in older adults. A nationwide survey conducted by the Centers for Disease Control and Prevention estimated an overall hypertension prevalence of 45% for American adults, with that prevalence rising to 75% for adults of age 60 and over.[1] While hypertension remains a growing concern in the geriatric population as a whole, racial and ethnic disparities in prevalence continue to persist. Non-Hispanic black (henceforth, black) adults have a higher prevalence of hypertension (57%) when compared to

[a] Division of Cardiology, Hypertension Section, Department of Internal Medicine, University of Texas Southwestern Medical Center, 5323 Harry Hines Boulevard B6.102, Dallas, TX 75390-9112, USA; [b] Division of Cardiology, Department of Internal Medicine, University of Texas Southwestern Medical Center, 5323 Harry Hines Boulevard B6.102, Dallas, TX 75390-9112, USA
* Corresponding author.
E-mail address: Shawna.Nesbitt@utsouthwestern.edu

Clin Geriatr Med 40 (2024) 529–538
https://doi.org/10.1016/j.cger.2024.04.010
0749-0690/24/© 2024 Elsevier Inc. All rights reserved.

non-Hispanic white (henceforth, white) adults (44%) and Hispanic adults (44%), across the continuum of age.[1,2] Over time, trends in hypertension also differ by race. From 1999 to 2016, the age-standardized prevalence of hypertension decreased among white adults, but not among Mexican American or black adults.[2]

Various social, economic, and environmental factors may account for the observed prevalence disparities in hypertension among older adults. Adequate nutrition with a diet high in fruits, vegetables, and low-fat dairy products has been demonstrated to lower blood pressure in individuals with and without hypertension.[3] Older blacks and Hispanics do not meet the daily requirement for fruits and vegetables, and blacks consume significantly less than Hispanics.[4]

Notable racial and ethnic disparities exist with respect to appropriate treatment of hypertension in older adults. Large, randomized trials have demonstrated clear benefits of appropriate blood pressure control in hypertensive older adults,[5,6] but treatment has not been consistently equitable among racial and ethnic groups.[7] A large analysis of over 16,000 participants in the National Health and Nutrition Examination Survey (NHANES) demonstrated that awareness, treatment, and control of hypertension were lower for black and Hispanic individuals relative to their white counterparts.[7] Additionally, when compared to white individuals, black individuals are diagnosed with hypertension at a younger age and have lived with hypertension longer when they reach older age.[8] This ultimately results in significantly higher rates of fatal stoke, end-stage renal disease, and cardiovascular mortality in this group.[8,9] Racial and ethnic minority adults requiring institutionalized or nursing home care receive fewer appropriate medical treatments, including preventive care, than white adults in the same setting.[10,11] Further, black and Hispanic older adults have less access to primary and specialty care overall and tend to receive less appropriate care when treated than white older adults.[12–14]

Perceptions and beliefs about hypertension clearly affect blood pressure treatment and control rates broadly and these beliefs often differ by race and ethnicity. A study of older persons showed that while blacks were more knowledgeable about the definition of hypertension and the relationship to kidney disease than whites or Hispanics, they were less likely to say that lifestyle modifications and alcohol reduction were effective in improving blood pressure control.[15] However, over time the misperceptions about hypertension among older black patients have shifted to be more aligned with clinical providers, yet the adherence to therapy is reflected by the degree to which older black patients understand the rationale for recommendations.[16]

Patient perceptions do not develop in isolation; years of discrimination in medicine have resulted in medical mistrust that leads to decreased health care utilization in minoritized older adults. Prior data suggest that most black and Hispanic patients in the United States believe the health care system treats people unfairly based on racial or ethnic background.[17] Unfortunately examples of mistreatment continue to occur. Individuals who harbor medical mistrust are less likely to seek medical care, keep follow-up appointments, and fill prescriptions, which, in patients with hypertension, can lead to suboptimal control.[18]

There is no doubt that disparities in the prevalence and the care of hypertension in older people continue to exist. Identifying contributors to these disparities is a critical step toward removing barriers to improve quality of life and outcomes (**Fig. 1**).

THE SOCIETAL CONTEXT OF RACIAL/ETHNIC OLDER ADULTS LIVING WITH HYPERTENSION

The underlying causes of the observed disparities in hypertension prevalence, diagnosis, treatment, and control are multifactorial. Although genetic polymorphisms

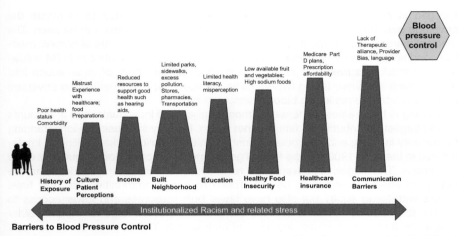

Barriers to Blood Pressure Control

Fig. 1. Older racial/ethnic minority persons experience multiple barriers to achieving blood pressure control. Institutionalized racism underlies most of these barriers and presents as a stressor.

explain some of the racial/ethnic differences in hypertension, the known contribution of genetic differences is quite small. Ignoring the vast differences in living circumstances between racial and ethnic groups effectively blinds health care providers to possible solutions that are in plain sight. Many disparities in hypertension are attributable to social and cultural differences.

Social determinants of health (SDOHs) are associated with increased mortality globally.[19] Older adults are more likely to have higher risk SDOHs, more physical limitations, and lower self-perception of good general health.[20] In a study of 954 older adults in the NHANES who self-rated their general health and functional limitations, older blacks had a significantly higher mean cumulative SDOH risk score (2.3 ± 2.1) compared to whites (1.5 ± 1.0). Among the risk factors assessed, educational attainment, poverty, food insecurity, and tobacco use were statistically significantly higher in prevalence among older blacks than whites. However, all risk factors trended higher in blacks.[21] Disproportionately limited access to care for minoritized older adults likely contributes to disparities in treatment and control of hypertension. Higher functional living limitations among black and Hispanic older adults impede their access to needed medical care.[22] The effect of SDOHs on health is the cumulative effect of a life-long exposure to these inequities that leads to significant disparities.[23]

Education level is associated with hypertension knowledge and control.[24] This relationship is unaffected by age. The racial/ethnic disparity in education is clear. Among US adults, 5.9% of whites, 11.9% of blacks, and 29.5% of Hispanics have less than a high school education. In older adults, the disparity in college education is even more evident with whites at 41.5%, blacks at 25.2%, and Hispanics at 19.5%.[25] Although hypertension knowledge is generally higher in Blacks, maintaining a focus on instruction at the level of the patient is an important component of reducing the disparity in hypertension.

Among older persons, Medicare is the most common form of insurance coverage. The implementation of changes to Medicare Part D was targeted to improve medication access and utilization. Despite overall improvements, the gap in coverage (known as the donut hole) led to more disparities in hypertensive medication use, as Hispanics and blacks were more likely to discontinue the use of medications when they reached the gap in coverage.[26] The Affordable Care Act was intended to eliminate the coverage gap, but the effects on disparities in older patients remain to be seen. The medical therapy management (MTM) program has improved the care of chronic medical conditions for some individuals; however, racial/ethnic disparities in MTM utilization and outcomes remain.[27] In 2015 to 2018%, 82% to 86% of older adults had hypertension and were taking hypertensive medications; thus, medication coverage is very important to achieving blood pressure control.[28]

Housing is the greatest expense for most families and individuals, and it accounts for the largest contribution to financial net worth. Inequity in housing is longstanding for minority families, and it is rooted in institutionalized policies like "redlining" implemented in the early 1900s by the federal government to protect home equity for white Americans. This largely disadvantaged minority communities for decades, and the long-term effects continue to persist. These redlined communities not only have homes with lower equity but also have fewer built resources and lower access to healthy food outlets.[29] This is perhaps the greatest disadvantage for minority older people, as their homes determine most of their wealth. The 2019 median income of households of older persons was $70,254; however, for whites, it was $74,365, $76,235 for Asians, $50,553 for Hispanics, and $51,743 for blacks. Among older people, 18% of blacks and 17.1% of Hispanics live below the poverty line. Most disturbing is that the highest poverty rates are found in older Hispanic women (32.1%) and older black women (31.7%).[28] While poverty influences the prevalence of hypertension in older adults, disparities that come with being black have a greater effect. Whereas poor white older adults living in poor white neighborhoods have higher prevalence of hypertension than poor whites living in non-poor white neighborhoods, blacks have higher prevalence of hypertension regardless of income or neighborhood.[30] Thus, race notably impacts hypertension prevalence of older persons.

Hidden in plain sight is the inequity in healthy food availability for communities of color. Across the United States, individuals who reside in areas of low socioeconomic housing suffer a second blow to their health with limited options for fresh foods. Black and Hispanic individuals have a higher likelihood of food insecurity in the United States compared to their white counterparts, which contributes to increased risk of obesity and resulting hypertension in these groups.[31,32] This is in part a carryover of the "redlining" policies of the past. Individuals living in food deserts are more likely to have hypertension and other cardiovascular risk factors; however, this relationship is amplified by household income, which tends to be lower in these areas.[33] In a cohort of older adults living in a food-insecure environment, the load of biomarkers of physiologic dysregulation is higher than in people living in food-secure areas. Importantly, the relationship is attenuated in individuals who participate in the Supplemental Nutrition Assistance Program.[34] Addressing the problem of unhealthy diets requires a complete understanding of the available food sources and the support available to individuals. Furthermore, large-scale efforts must be made on regional and national levels to ensure equitable nutrition for minoritized groups.

Although the immediate effect of nicotine on blood pressure is short-lived, the relationship between nicotine use and poor cardiovascular outcomes is well established. Efforts to curtail smoking between 2011 and 2022 have been largely positive in all age groups except in older adults. Smoking rates in older adults have remained at 10% in this period. Older persons living 200% below the poverty level have higher smoking prevalence than higher income persons.[35] Disparities in smoking behavior show that African Americans are more likely to smoke menthol cigarettes, and sadly menthol smokers have lower rates of success with smoking cessation.[36] Furthermore, smoking is more common among older blacks with hypertension than whites.[37] Interestingly, menthol cigarettes are more frequently marketed in poor and black neighborhoods.[38] Public health messaging is needed to inform individuals of this systematic targeting by retailers.

The effect of one's culture on health is significant. Life expectancy among Hispanics is similar to that of whites, despite having lower access to housing, education, income, and health care. This paradox is thought to be related to the cultural practice of "familism," which values caring for family members.[39] In focus group studies of black hypertensive patients, social support, positive health care experiences, and family-centered values enhanced self-management of hypertension. Alternatively, family habits and feelings about illness and food traditions tended hinder self-management of blood pressure.[40] The "circle of culture," or that which connects individuals to other individuals within a culture, has a powerful effect on acceptance of interventions such as dietary changes. This acceptance is important to mitigate the alienation and isolation that black individuals feel in the larger culture of the United States.[41] Among older persons, social connection is important to protect health-related quality of life. The diversity of the social network is more significant than the perceived quality of the social support.[42] Improving the care of hypertensive older persons should include an assessment of the social environment and the family support for racial and ethnic minority patients to improve health equity in hypertension.

SOLUTIONS

The approach to reducing disparities in hypertension in older persons is as broad as the factors that contribute to their presence. Each entity must take on a responsibility for mitigating the barrier in their sphere of influence.

Health care systems are charged with a duty to assess the quality, safety, and equity of the care they provide. They regularly review the data in their system as a matter of usual business and quality control. An assessment of the SDOHs is just the starting point to understanding the needs of individual patients and the background they come from. The electronic health record is a conduit for accessing this information, but the information must be carefully collected by trained individuals with a deliberate approach to capture information accurately and sensitively. These data are only as good as the method used to collect it. Data from large systems can be useful in defining targeted approaches to the disparities in the national and local community.[43] Health care systems have the power to address local disparities in hypertension through leveraging relationships with local businesses and nonprofit organizations. The strength of this approach is found in the personal connection and a more specific intervention in the communities that they collectively serve.

Health care insurance is only one component in access to care. While Medicare largely resolves issues of hospital visits and clinic visits, Medicare Part D has not yet eliminated the disparity in access to medications. Continuing to deliver health care as a "privilege' rather than a right of all members of society perpetuates the inequity in health care. Beyond insurance, access to care is also affected by the distance and location of services to individuals from minority communities. Health care is "local" and as such, city planners and health care systems must think of innovative ideas such as "medical malls" to address the limitation in locations of health care facilities and providers to ensure that patients truly have equal access.[44]

Blood pressure screenings that are conducted in older persons from minority groups are another method of reducing health disparities in blood pressure control. The frequent variation in blood pressure and orthostasis among older persons increases the risk of events. Screening blood pressures and home blood pressures are helpful in directing appropriate therapy. Community screening events offer another opportunity to promote proper blood pressure technique and education on hypertension outside of the clinical environment.[45]

The role of physicians in promoting health equity is embedded in the Hippocratic oath "to do no harm" and the American Medical Association Code of Ethics which recognizes the responsibility of physicians to contribute to the betterment of public health and the improvement of the community.[46] Practicing "cultural humility" is a practical approach to learning about patient experiences and cultural backgrounds. This can have major implications into patient responses to therapeutic decisions. Many dimensions of hypertensive care of racial/ethnic minority patients are affected by their social and cultural circumstances. Lifestyle modification recommendations are affected by the built environment patients live in. Understanding patients' perceptions about health care providers and medications may help to facilitate a more transparent and realistic conversation regarding treatments for blood pressure. Multiple studies of medication adherence in black patients with hypertension show that "therapeutic alliance"–based interventions that rely on the collaborative bond between patients and providers effectively improve adherence to therapy in this population.[47] Furthermore, physicians have a unique view of the barriers that hinder patients and drive disparities in hypertension. In patient interactions, ensuring that patients understand instructions and agree that they are feasible to follow is a key component to improving control rates. Both sides of the communication gap must be addressed from low health and digital literacy and limited English proficiency in patients to low cultural humility, unconscious bias, and inexperience with shared decision-making in providers.[48] Furthermore, providers should adjust instructions to fit with the cultural background befitting to the patient. Physicians are the 'eyes and ears' of society on health disparities. This role extends beyond observation and reporting but rather interpreting for society the specific needs to be addressed to achieve greater equity (**Table 1**).

Table 1 What providers can do to help older patients overcome barriers to blood pressure control	
	Description
Implicit bias	Reflect on your implicit bias; practice cultural humility.
Know your local neighborhoods	Get to know the local environment and neighborhood patients live in.
Assess social determinant information	Implement a method of understanding your patients social determinants of health in a sensitive and accurate manner.
Knowledge of available local and national resources	Provide resources for patients to become familiar with available resources for healthy food and other support.
Practice therapeutic alliance in treatment	Engage patients in decisions about therapeutic choices.
Understand family and support system	Engage the support network in treatment plan.
Advocate for patients	Advocate for patients needs based on your direct experience with patients for systematic changes to support health equity.
Ensure good communication with patients	Assess their comprehension of instructions, language proficiency, assess health literacy and meet patient where they are.
Culture and perceptions	Ask patients about their practices at home and thoughts about health care.

The role of government and community organizations in resolving disparities in hypertension is broad. Addressing the needs of housing and the built environment to promote healthy living lies squarely in their control. Living in neighborhoods that lack walkable sidewalks, safe parks and recreation, safe locations for community gatherings, accessible and affordable healthy foods, and safe forms of transportation is a limitation for older persons to live healthy lower stress lives that facilitate better blood pressure control.

Racism underlies many of the disparities in hypertension and other illnesses. Many of the conditions cast as problems for underprivileged persons are a manifestation of institutionalized racism. Practices such as redlining may no longer be legal, but the effects of these early policies remain in place. To rectify this, these effects must be acknowledged to facilitate solutions that resonate throughout many of the SDOHs that impede equity in blood pressure control.

SUMMARY

Hypertension is a significant health concern in older persons and its contribution to morbidity, quality of life, and mortality in older persons from minority racial and ethnic backgrounds is unacceptable. To remedy this inequity, the search for solutions must include a complete assessment of the social, racial, and cultural factors that are embedded in the problem. Bringing these issues to the forefront can be accomplished best with the inclusion of voices from broad backgrounds and perspectives.

CLINICS CARE POINTS

- Focus on strong communication with patients.
- Collect information on social determinants of health and facilitate connection to resources to address issues.
- Educate clinical staff on the local environment and community needs of the patient population.

DISCLOSURES

S. D. Nesbitt, MD, MS, serves as a site principal investigator for a clinical trial sponsored by Ablative Solutions. S. V. Carter has nothing to disclose.

REFERENCES

1. Ostchega Y, Fryar CD, Nwankwo T, et al. Hypertension Prevalence among adults aged 18 and over: United States, 2017-2018. NCHS Data Brief 2020;364:1–8.
2. Dorans KS, Mills KT, Liu Y, et al. Trends in prevalence and control of hypertension according to the 2017 American College of Cardiology/American Heart Association (ACC/AHA) Guideline. J Am Heart Assoc 2018;7(11):e00888.
3. Sacks FM, Svetkey LP, Vollmer WM, et al. Effects on blood pressure of reduced dietary sodium and the dietary approaches to stop hypertension (DASH) diet. DASH-sodium collaborative research group. N Engl J Med 2001;344(1):3–10.
4. Kibe LW, Bazargan M. Fruit and vegetable intake among older African American and hispanic adults with cardiovascular risk factors. Gerontol Geriatr Med 2022; 8:23337214211057730.

5. Beckett NS, Peters R, Fletcher AE, et al. Treatment of hypertension in patients 80 years of age or older. N Engl J Med 2008;358(18):1887–98.
6. Williamson JD, Supiano MA, Applegate WB, et al. Intensive vs standard blood pressure control and cardiovascular disease outcomes in adults aged ≥75 Years: a randomized clinical trial. JAMA 2016;315(24):2673–82.
7. Aggarwal R, Chiu N, Wadhera RK, et al. Racial/ethnic disparities in hypertension prevalence, awareness, treatment, and control in the United States, 2013 to 2018. Hypertension 2021;78(6):1719–26.
8. Hardy ST, Chen L, Cherrington AL, et al. Racial and ethnic differences in blood pressure among US adults, 1999-2018. Hypertension 2021;78(6):1730–41.
9. Ferdinand KC, Armani AM. The management of hypertension in African Americans. Crit Pathw Cardiol 2007;6(2):67–71.
10. Allsworth JE, Toppa R, Palin NC, et al. Racial and ethnic disparities in the pharmacologic management of diabetes mellitus among long-term care facility residents. Ethn Dis 2005;15(2):205–12.
11. Travers JL, Schroeder KL, Blaylock TE, et al. Racial/ethnic disparities in influenza and pneumococcal vaccinations among nursing home residents: a systematic review. Gerontol 2018;58(4):e205–17.
12. Mahmoudi E, Jensen GA. Exploring disparities in access to physician services among older adults: 2000-2007. J Gerontol B Psychol Sci Soc Sci 2013;68(1): 128–38.
13. Blustein J, Weiss LJ. Visits to specialists under Medicare: socioeconomic advantage and access to care. J Health Care Poor Underserved 1998;9(2):153–69.
14. McBean AM, Gornick M. Differences by race in the rates of procedures performed in hospitals for Medicare beneficiaries. Health Care Financ Rev 1994; 15(4):77–90.
15. Okonofua EC, Cutler NE, Lackland DT, et al. Ethnic differences in older americans: awareness, knowledge, and beliefs about hypertension. Am J Hypertens 2005;18(7):972–9.
16. Buckley L, Labonville S, Barr J. A systematic review of beliefs about hypertension and its treatment among African Americans. Curr Hypertens Rep 2016;18(7):52.
17. Fletcher M. Black Americans see a health-care system infected by racism, new poll shows. National Geographic History & Culture. Washington, DC: National Geographic Society; 2020.
18. LaVeist TA, Isaac LA, Williams KP. Mistrust of health care organizations is associated with underutilization of health services. Health Serv Res 2009;44(6): 2093–105.
19. Marmot M. Social determinants of health inequities. Lancet 2005;365:1009–104.
20. Rhee TG, Marttoli RA, Cooney LM, et al. Associations of social and behavioral determinants of health index with self-rated health, functional limitations, and health services use in older adults. J Am Geriatr Soc 2020;68:1731–8.
21. Rhee TG, Lee K, Schensul S. Black-White disparities in social and behavioral determinants of health index and their associations with self-rated health and functional limitations in older adults. J Gerontol A Biol Sci Med Sci 2021;76(4):735–40.
22. Travers JL, D'Arpino S, Bradway C, et al. Minority older adults' access to and use of programs of all-inclusive care for the elderly. J Aging Soc Policy 2022;34(6): 976–1002.
23. Marmot M. Just societies, health equity, and dignified lives: the PAHO equity commission. Lancet 2018;392:2247–50.
24. Oliveria SA, Chen RS, McCarthy BD, et al. Hypertension knowledge, awareness, and attitudes in a hypertensive population. J Gen Intern Med 2005;20:219–25.

25. Taylor M, Turk JM, Chessman HM, and Espinosa LL. Race and Ethnicity in Higher Education: A Status Report, 2020 Supplement. Published by American Council on Education Supported by the Andrew Mellon Foundation. Available at: www.equityinhighered.org.

26. Zissimopoulos J, Joyce GF, Scarpati LM, et al. Did Medicare Part D reduce disparities? Am J Manag Care 2015;21(2):119–28.

27. Dong X, Tsang CCS, Browning JA, et al. Racial and Ethnic Disparities in Medicare Part D medication therapy management services utilization. Exploratory Research in Clinical and Social Pharmacy 2023;9:100222.

28. The 2021 Profile of Older Americans. 2022. The Administration for Community Living, which includes the Administration on Aging, a division of the U.S, Department of Health and Human Services.

29. McClure E, Feinstein L, Cordoba E, et al. The legacy of redlining in the effect of foreclosures on Detroit residents' self-rated health. Health Place 2019;55:9–19.

30. Usher T, Gaskin DJ, Bower K, et al. Residential segregation and hypertension prevalence in Black and white older adults. J Appl Gerontol 2018;37(2):177–202.

31. Brandt EJ, Chang T, Leung C, et al. Food insecurity among individuals with cardiovascular disease and cardiometabolic risk factors across race and ethnicity in 1999-2018. JAMA Cardiol 2022;7(12):1218–26.

32. Testa A, Jackson DB. Food insecurity, food deserts, and waist-to-height ratio: variation by sex and race/ethnicity. J Community Health 2019;44(3):444–50.

33. Kelli HM, Hammadah M, Ahmed H, et al. Association between living in food deserts and cardiovascular risk. Circ Cardiovasc Qual Outcomes 2017;10(9): e003532.

34. Pak TY, Kim G. Association of food insecurity with allostatic load among older adults in the US. JAMA Netw Open 2021;4(12):e2137503.

35. Meza R, Cao P, Jeon J, et al. Trends in US adult smoking prevalence, 2011 to 2022. JAMA Health Forum 2023;4(12):e234213.

36. Jones JT, Xu K, Deng L, et al. Smoking cessation prevalence by menthol cigarette use and select demographics among adults in the United States, TUS-CPS, 2003-2019. Prev Med Rep 2023;36:102440.

37. Egan BM, Bland VJ, Brown AL, et al. Hypertension in african americans aged 60 to 79 years: statement from the international society of hypertension in blacks. J Clin Hypertens 2015;17(4):252–9.

38. Mills SD, Henriksen L, Golden SD, et al. Disparities in retail marketing for menthol cigarettes in the United States, 2015. Health Place 2018;53:62–70.

39. Perez FP, Perez C, Chumbiauca MN. Insights into social determinants of health in older adults. J Biomed Sci Eng 2022;15(11):261–8.

40. Long E, Ponder M, Bernard S. Knowledge, attitudes, and beliefs related to hypertension and hyperlipidemia self-management among African American men living in the southeastern United States. Patient Educ Couns 2017;100(5):1000–6.

41. Peters RM, Aroian KJ, Flack JM. African American culture and hypertension prevention. West J Nurs Res 2006;28(7):831–54 ; discussion 855-63.

42. Rhee TG, Marottoli RA, Monin JK. Diversity of social networks versus quality of social support: which is more protective for health-related quality of life among older adults? Prev Med 2021;145:106440.

43. Angier H, Huguet N, Marino M, et al. Observational study protocol for evaluating control of hypertension and the effects of social determinants. BMJ Open 2019; 9(3):e025975.

44. Ito A. Medical mall founders' satisfaction and integrated management requirements. Int J Health Plann Manage 2017;32(4):449–64.

45. Anker D, Santos-Eggimann B, Santschi V, et al. Screening and treatment of hypertension in older adults: less is more? Public Health Rev 2018;39:26.
46. Bryan CS. What is the oslerian tradition? Ann Intern Med 1994;120:682.
47. Desta R, Blumrosen C, Laferriere HE, et al. Interventions incorporating therapeutic alliance to improve medication adherence in Black patients with diabetes, hypertension and kidney disease: a systematic review. Patient Prefer Adherence 2022;16:3095–110.
48. Pérez-Stable EJ, El-Toukhy S. Communicating with diverse patients: how patient and clinician factors affect disparities. Patient Educ Couns 2018;101(12): 2186–94.

The Role of Vascular Aging in the Development of Hypertension

Celia Pena Heredia, MD[a], Deborah Furman, MD[a,1],
Denisse G. Moreno, MD[b,2], Eric Tuday, MD, PhD[c,d,e,3,*]

KEYWORDS

- Vascular stiffness • Older adult • Hypertension • Cellular senescence • Senolytics

KEY POINTS

- Vascular stiffness increases with age and is intimately associated with hypertension and other comorbidities seen in older adults and is also as an independent risk factor for predicting cardiovascular morbidity and mortality.
- Vascular stiffness can be readily measured and quantified in a clinical setting in an independent manner using relatively fast, non-invasive methods in a clinic setting.
- Therapeutics are currently limited to treat vascular stiffness; however, there are promising approaches on the horizon that encompass both pharmacologic and non-pharmacologic methods.

INTRODUCTION

In older adults, vascular stiffness has been shown to be an independent predictor of cardiovascular (CV) morbidity and mortality.[1,2] It has been shown that vascular stiffness increases proportionally with age and that increased vascular stiffness with aging has been closely associated with the development of isolated systolic hypertension

Funding sources for all authors: E. Tuday is supported by the National Institutes of Health, United States Awards, K08 AG070281 and the Western Institute for Veterans Research. D.G. Moreno is supported by T32HL139451.
a Department of Internal Medicine, University of Utah; b Division of Geriatrics, Department of Internal Medicine, University of Utah; c Division of Cardiology, Department of Internal Medicine, University of Utah, 30 Mario Capecchi Drive, Salt Lake City, UT 84112, USA; d Salt Lake City Veterans Affairs Hospital; e Geriatrics Research Education and Clinical Center (GRECC)
1 Present address: 830 East 6th Avenue, Apartment 12, Salt Lake City, UT 84103.
2 Present address: 1350 East 4750 South Apartment E9, Salt Lake City, UT 84117.
3 Present address: 4493 South Parkview Drive, Salt Lake City, UT 84124.
* Corresponding author. HELIX Building Level 3; 30 North Mario Capecchi Drive, Salt Lake City, UT 84112.
E-mail address: Eric.Tuday@hsc.utah.edu
Twitter: @debfurman_MD (D.F.); @DenisseG_Moreno (D.G.M.)

Clin Geriatr Med 40 (2024) 539–550
https://doi.org/10.1016/j.cger.2024.04.011
geriatric.theclinics.com

(HTN).[2–4] From a hemodynamic standpoint, with a stiffer, more rigid vascular wall comes a higher systolic pressure within the vasculature during each cardiac cycle, for a given stroke volume. While the development of HTN with aging is multifactorial with involvement of multiple organ systems, due to the innate relationship between vascular health and blood pressure (BP), a closer review of vascular health and stiffness is warranted.

CELLULAR CHANGES IN THE DEVELOPMENT OF VASCULAR STIFFNESS

It is has been well documented that age-related changes in the vasculature—including endothelial dysfunction, increased extracellular fibrosis, and an increased burden of senescent (a state of nonproliferation, dysfunction, and inflammatory/fibrotic molecule secretion), endothelial and smooth muscle cells are associated with increased vascular stiffness with aging.[5–7] While endothelial cell dysfunction and extracellular fibrosis have been reviewed in detail, cellular senescence and its role in vascular function and stiffness have emerged in the past 5 to 10 years. [5–7]

With aging, endothelial cells, smooth muscle cells, and fibroblasts enter a senescent state where they undergo cell cycle arrest and develop a senescence-associated secretory phenotype (SASP). Cellular senescence is typically a product of aging; however, exposure to increased levels of reactive oxygen species and DNA damage can induce premature cellular senescence.[8] While the onset of cellular senescence may be viewed as beneficial in certain proliferative disorders, such as oncologic diseases, there is growing consensus that a high burden of senescent cells within a particular organ is relatively detrimental.[9] The SASP profile for a particular cell and organ system is often specific in terms of molecules but is typically both proinflammatory and profibrotic.[9,10] The SASP of the vasculature has been well described and generally consists of inflammatory cytokines (eg, IL-6, IL-1β, TNFα) and proteases which lead to fibrosis and inflammation of the vascular wall through collagen deposition, elastin degradation, and cross linking of structural proteins by advanced glycation end products.[5,11,12] Senescent cells, particularly vascular endothelial cells, have recently been linked to increased vascular stiffness in animals.[5]

EPIDEMIOLOGY OF VASCULAR STIFFNESS

In general, vascular stiffness increases with age in the general population.[13,14] Women tend to have accelerated vascular stiffening later in life and older women typically have higher vascular stiffness when compared to older men.[15–18] Few studies have focused on the ethnoracial differences affecting arterial stiffness in the geriatric population. **Table 1** summarizes the pertinent details of these studies. Overall, vascular stiffness almost universally increases with age to some degree and the most robust ethnic-specific comparison that has held across studies is that people of African descent typically have a higher vascular stiffness at a given age when compared to white populations.[19–23]

THE ROLE OF VASCULAR STIFFNESS IN CARDIOVASCULAR DISEASE

The most direct sequela of increased vascular stiffness is the development of isolated systolic HTN.[24] Increased arterial stiffness results in augmented impedance of the aorta and decreased arterial compliance, which causes higher systolic blood pressure (SBP) and an increase in pulse wave velocity (PWV; a measure of vascular stiffness).[25] Details of the PWV measurement will follow. In brief, pulse waves are transmitted more rapidly in stiffer central arterial systems. In serial studies using 4 dimensional MRI,

Table 1
Studies describing differences in arterial stiffness in older populations

Reference, Country	Age (Years), Ethnicity	N	Arterial Stiffness (P<0.05*)	Device	Additional Comments
Brar et al,[20] 2020; Canada	South Asian: 71 ± 5; White: 71 ± 5	South Asian: 22; White: 22	baPWV (m/s) South Asian: 12 ± 2; White: 11 ±2 CC (mm²/kPa) South Asian: 0.6 ± 0.3; White: 0.8 ± 0.3*	Pulse Transducer, ADInstruments; Doppler Ultrasound, Compumedics CC obtained from PP measurement of the CCA by applanation tonometry, Millar Instruments.	38.6% of the participants had HTN.
Guo et al,[21] 2016; China and Sweden	Swedish: 72.5 ± 5.5; Chinese: 75 ± 6.5	Swedish: 3049; Chinese: 1272	cfPWV (m/s) Swedish: 10.1 (8.8–11.8)*; Chinese 8.9 (7.6–10.5)	Applanation Tonometry, SphygmoCor.	70.2% of Swedish and 70.1% of the Chinese participants had HTN, while 5.2% of Swedish and 6.7% of Chinese participants had DM.
Markert et al,[22] 2020; United States	Black: 72 ±9; White: 74 ±9; Hispanic: 68 ±8	Black: 317; White: 271; Hispanic: 948	Carotid stiffness Black: 9.24 ±6.21*; White: 8.74 ±6.91; Hispanic: 8.40 ± 5.65	Carotid stiffness derived from carotid intraluminal diameters and brachial blood pressure. Carotid US data via GE LOGIQ system. Blood pressure via Dinamap Pro100.	70% of participants had HTN (Black 76%, White 61%, Hispanic 70%) and 19% had DM (Black 21%, White 9%, Hispanic 21%).

(continued on next page)

Table 1
(continued)

Reference, Country	Age (Years), Ethnicity	N	Arterial Stiffness (P<0.05*)	Device	Additional Comments
Park et al,[23] 2011; England	African Caribbean: 70.1 ±5.9; European: 69.7 ± 6.2; South Asian: 69.0 ± 6.1	African Caribbean: 169; European: 442; South Asian: 349	cfPWV (m/s) ([mean ± SE]) African Caribbean: 10.9 ±0.02; European: 11.5 ± 0.01; South Asian: 11.3 ± 0.01	cfPWV measured using Doppler probe Central hemodynamics via SphygmoCor	79% of Black, 57% of White and 75% of South Asian participants had HTN, while 41% of Black, 19% of White and 41% of South Asian participants had DM.

Table based on the epidemiology review by Schutte and colleagues.[19] Data are mean ± SD unless otherwise specified. White refers to Caucasian individuals and Black refers to individuals of African descent. The * refers to the studies below in the column that have met the statistical significance of $P<0.05$.

Abbreviations: baPWV, brachial-ankle PWV; CC, compliance coefficient; CCA, common carotid artery; cfPWV, carotid–femoral PWV; DM, diabetes mellitus; HTN, hypertension; PP, pulse pressure.

older groups (70–80 years of age) of men and women experienced higher increases of PWV compared to younger subjects when followed for 6 years.[26] Older patients (68 ± 6 years) with isolated systolic HTN have higher aortic PWV and impaired endothelial function when compared to age-matched healthy controls.[3] The long-term consequences of uncontrolled HTN are clear in terms of morbidity and mortality.

ASSOCIATED VASCULAR STIFFNESS COMORBIDITIES

While increased vascular stiffness is an independent predictor of CV morbidity and mortality, it has also been implicated in the pathophysiology of disease of other organ systems.[27] The exact mechanism has not fully been elucidated and is probably different for each organ system, but one leading hypothesis is that altered hemodynamics and greater perfusion pulsatile pressures lead to damage of the vascular bed (**Fig. 1**).[27] Increased vascular stiffness has been implicated in diastolic dysfunction and heart failure, chronic kidney disease (CKD), and even cognitive dysfunction (see **Fig. 1**).[27]

Diastolic dysfunction, as measured by echocardiography, is significantly associated with increased vascular stiffness.[28–30] Furthermore, studies have shown that the presence of increased vascular stiffness is associated with new onset heart failure with preserved ejection fraction (HFpEF).[28,30,31] It is thought that the aortic stiffness increases seen after age of 50 years leads to increases in afterload on the left ventricle (LV) and causes the LV remodeling, hypertrophy, and diastolic dysfunction.[32,33] The progression of LV diastolic dysfunction is likely a key factor for the development of HFpEF.[14,28–31]

Regarding the relationship of vascular stiffness and CKD, studies have shown that increased aortic PWV correlates with decreased creatinine clearance in both hypertensive and normotensive subjects.[34] Zuo and colleagues showed that compared

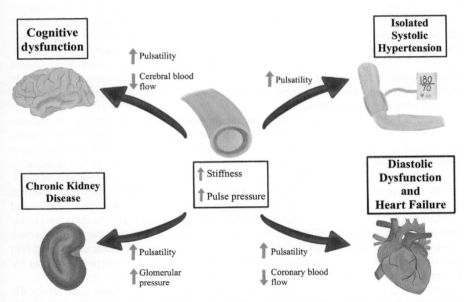

Fig. 1. The mechanical effect of increased vascular stiffness leading to increased pulse wave pulsatility in end-organs vascular beds and proposed mechanisms of contribution to end-organ damage and chronic disease.

with HTN without CKD, hypertensive patients with CKD have higher carotid–femoral PWV and intima–media thickness measured by ultrasound.[35] More recently, Tian and colleagues were able to establish a causal relationship between increased PWV and CKD in a large population in northern China.[36] As Insierra and colleagues have reviewed, this is a 2 way pathway in which the vascular inflammation enhanced by CKD promotes vascular stiffness by stimulating fibrosis and proliferation of the vascular smooth muscle cells.[37]

Lastly, the observations of vascular stiffness in cognitive dysfunction are interesting. In the Maine-Syracuse Longitudinal Study, Elias and colleagues discovered that the combination of higher PWV and older age resulted in progressively lower cognitive performance in a battery of tests.[38] Similar results were drawn out by the Baltimore Longitudinal Study of Aging[39] and from a prospective study of older French patients with subjective memory complaints.[40] In a group of older Americans (45% Black, 27% with mild cognitive impairment), Hugues and colleagues found that an increased PWV measured in a central vascular bed, was associated with greater cortical β-amyloid deposition measured by PET, lower brain volumes in Alzheimer disease—susceptible regions and high white matter hyperintensity burden measured by MRI. These associations were independent of *APOE* ε4 status.[41] In the Framingham Offspring Study, higher carotid–femoral PWV was associated with greater white matter hyperintensity volume ($P=0.005$) and lower total cerebral brain volume ($P=0.02$).[42]

MEASURING VASCULAR STIFFNESS

There are several clinical measures to indirectly assess central and peripheral arterial stiffness. The simplest proxy for central arterial stiffness is the pulse pressure—the delta between SBP and diastolic BP measurements. To truly measure intrinsic vascular stiffness, one currently would need to perform mechanical testing in an ex vivo manner. This is clearly not feasible in a clinical setting, and as such, methods have been developed that represent the degree of vascular stiffness present. The gold standard for assessing vascular stiffness, noninvasively, has traditionally been through the use of pressure tonometry and ultrasound imaging to generate objective measures.[43–45] These measurements: PWV, arterial distensibility, and peripheral arterial pressure waveform analysis; were discussed in detail in the prior issue in Clinics in Geriatric Medicine and will be briefly reviewed here.[46] Newer, noninvasive methods are currently in development.

Vascular PWV measurements have historically been used as an indicator of vascular stiffness. With each heart beat, a pressure wave is generated in the proximal aorta which then propagates throughout the arterial tree. The speed of the pressure wave is directly related to the stiffness of the vessel (ie, a higher vascular stiffness equates to a higher PWV). Initially, PWV was measured via intravascular measurements obtained by pressure wire catheters. However, the most common noninvasive method is by use of pressure tonography, measuring the mechanical distension of the vessel in a carotid–femoral (cf) or brachial–ankle (ba) pairing. By pairing these data with time-gated electrocardiogram (EKG) and the physical distance between the measurement sites, one is able to derive vascular PWV. In a similar manner, vascular ultrasound can be implemented to detect the pressure/flow wave via Doppler imaging, allowing for the collection of similar data with albeit a large equipment footprint.

Lastly, new computation techniques and imaging algorithms have allowed for 4D vessel flow (time-resolved 3D volumetric flow) calculations utilizing MRI.[47–49] The measurements have been shown to be highly accurate and allows for local and global assessments of vascular stiffness with the pitfalls being the cost and availability of MRI.

Arterial distensibility and peripheral arterial pressure waveform analysis are both important measures of vascular mechanics but are not commonly utilized or referenced in a clinical setting.[50,51] Arterial distensibility measures the response of the arterial diameter to that of a given pulse pressure (the difference between SBP and diastolic BP) where decreased distensibility is suggestive of increased vascular stiffness. These measures are typically made via pressure tonometry and reflect site-specific conditions. However, noninvasive imaging such as cardiac computed tomography (CT) or MRI can allow for central aorta distensibility measurements when combined with accurate real-time BP monitoring.[52] Lastly, an indicator that a patient may have increased vascular stiffness is the presence of aortic calcium as determined by CT scanning, as studies have shown its presence is significantly associated with higher PWVs.[53]

MODULATING VASCULAR STIFFNESS
Pharmacologic Therapy

While measures of vascular stiffness generally show improvement with treatment of BP, the goal of obtaining a therapy that specifically targets mechanical properties of the vasculature to help promote positive remodeling with a reduction of stiffness remains largely unmet.[54] To date, pharmacologic therapy that independently affects vascular stiffness outside of BP lowering has not been promising. Agents that target the renin–angiotensin–aldosterone system seem to have the most promise, showing in some meta-analyses the decrease in vascular stiffness beyond their BP effect; however, the data remain somewhat mixed. [54–58] The effects of statins on vascular stiffness have been inconsistently studied, with mostly smaller trials; however, statins do appear to at a minimum prevent progression of vascular stiffness and may act to improve it through BP independent mechanisms.[10,54,59,60] Lastly, on the horizon is the potential use of senolytic therapy (agents that specifically target and clear senescent cells). The use these agents have shown benefit in treating vascular stiffness in animals.[5] The use of senolytic agents in humans has only just entered into clinical trials with the first trial focusing on treatment of idiopathic pulmonary fibrosis.[61,62]

Non-pharmacologic Therapy

Non-pharmacological management of arterial stiffness remains an ongoing area of study. The vasodilatory effect of heat in the setting of thermoregulation is well studied. Recently, attention has been directed toward the acute effects of warm water immersion (WWI) on vascular stiffness as measured by PWV. Sugawara and colleagues saw a modest reduction in PWV immediately following WWI in a small sample; however, it is unknown whether the protective benefit is lasting.[63] Upon exposure to cold, blood vessels constrict, reducing compliance in a physiologic response to preserve core body temperature. However, emerging evidence has demonstrated a longitudinal benefit of cold exposure on vascular aging. Forthcoming research has demonstrated a reduction in medial arterial calcification and senescence in mice when exposed to cold temperatures.[64]

Exercise and diet have endured as the cornerstone of non-pharmacological therapy of arterial stiffness. The benefit of exercise is multifaceted including strengthening of mitochondrial defense against exercise induced reactive oxidant species, which in turn leads to reduced oxidative damage in the vasculature. Additionally, studies show that exercise preserves endothelial functioning and reduces vascular inflammation.[65–67] Caloric restricted diets improve arterial stiffness by changing aortic distensibility and increasing endothelial nitric oxide synthases. Saturated fats, trans fats, cholesterol, and sucrose all contribute to worsening vascular stiffness. Thus, patients should be counseled on a diet that emphasizes fruits, vegetables, whole grains, and lean protein, while limiting saturated fats and complex carbohydrates with a high glycemic index to prevent vascular aging.[68] This dietary pattern shares many aspects of the Mediterranean diet and the DASH diet, two diets endorsed by the American Heart Association in the prevention of CV disease.[69] Lastly, a pure focus on dietary sodium reduction also appears to have, in part, a BP-independent impact on vascular stiffness according to a recent meta-analysis, where an average of a 2 g decrease in daily sodium intake resulted in a mild reduction in PWV. [70]

Many dietary patterns captivate a subset of the population due to their purported health benefits. In the past decade, intermittent fasting and the ketogenic diet have entered the vernacular as restrictive diets that can improve metabolic health, met with mixed scientific evidence.[71,72] While robust data are lacking, intermittent fasting has been shown to improve arterial stiffness and the ketogenic diet has been shown to worsen arterial stiffness.[73,74]

Recommendations for Monitoring Vascular Stiffness

Currently, guidelines do not provide a strong recommendation for the routine use and monitoring of vascular stiffness, partly due to the lack of specific, effective therapies that target vascular stiffness beyond the treatment of HTN. [57,75–78] Measurements of vascular stiffness can be made to help further risk stratify patients, especially if in shared decision making, there is uncertainty on whether to initiate a specific care plan.[57]

SUMMARY

Increased vascular stiffness with aging represents a significant health risk, both directly with the development of HTN, but also with disease processes in other organ systems.

CLINICS CARE POINTS

- Increased vascular stiffness with age has important implications in risk stratifying patients in terms of cardiovascular morbiditiy and mortality, especially playing a key role in the development of isolated systolic hypertension.
- New emerging pharamacologic and non-pharmacologic interventions are showing promise in terms of impacting vascular stiffness and clinicians should take this into consideration when assess and treating older patients with hypertension.

DISCLOSURE

E. Tuday is receiving an honorarium from Elsevier as a guest co-editor.

REFERENCES

1. Laurent S, Boutouyrie P, Asmar R, et al. Aortic stiffness is an independent predictor of all-cause and cardiovascular mortality in hypertensive patients. Hypertension 2001;37(5):1236–41.
2. Najjar SS, Scuteri A, Shetty V, et al. Pulse wave velocity is an independent predictor of the longitudinal increase in systolic blood pressure and of incident hypertension in the Baltimore Longitudinal Study of Aging. J Am Coll Cardiol 2008; 51(14):1377–83.

3. Wallace SM, Yasmin Mc, Eniery CM, et al. Isolated systolic hypertension is characterized by increased aortic stiffness and endothelial dysfunction. Hypertension 2007;50(1):228–33.
4. Boutouyrie P, Chowienczyk P, Humphrey JD, et al. Arterial stiffness and cardiovascular risk in hypertension. Circ Res 2021;128(7):864–86.
5. Clayton ZS, Rossman MJ, Mahoney SA, et al. Cellular senescence contributes to large elastic artery stiffening and endothelial dysfunction with aging: Amelioration with senolytic treatment. Hypertension 2023;80(10):2072–87.
6. Lakatta EG. Arterial and cardiac aging: major shareholders in cardiovascular disease enterprises: Part III: cellular and molecular clues to heart and arterial aging. Circulation 2003;107(3):490–7.
7. Ungvari Z, Tarantini S, Donato AJ, et al. Mechanisms of vascular aging. Circ Res 2018;123(7):849–67.
8. Zhu Y, Armstrong JL, Tchkonia T, et al. Cellular senescence and the senescent secretory phenotype in age-related chronic diseases. Curr Opin Clin Nutr Metab Care 2014;17(4):324–8.
9. Mylonas A, O'Loghlen A. Cellular senescence and ageing: mechanisms and interventions. Front Aging 2022;3:866718.
10. McHugh D, Gil J. Senescence and aging: causes, consequences, and therapeutic avenues. J Cell Biol 2018;217(1):65–77.
11. Gardner SE, Humphry M, Bennett MR, et al. Senescent vascular smooth muscle cells drive inflammation through an interleukin-1alpha-dependent senescence-associated secretory phenotype. Arterioscler Thromb Vasc Biol 2015;35(9):1963–74.
12. Han Y, Kim SY. Endothelial senescence in vascular diseases: current understanding and future opportunities in senotherapeutics. Exp Mol Med 2023;55(1):1–12.
13. Mitchell GF, Parise H, Benjamin EJ, et al. Changes in arterial stiffness and wave reflection with advancing age in healthy men and women: the Framingham Heart Study. Hypertension 2004;43(6):1239–45.
14. Redfield MM, Jacobsen SJ, Borlaug BA, et al. Age- and gender-related ventricular-vascular stiffening: a community-based study. Circulation 2005;112(15): 2254–62.
15. Russo C, Jin Z, Palmieri V, et al. Arterial stiffness and wave reflection. Hypertension 2012;60(2):362–8.
16. Coutinho T, Borlaug BA, Pellikka PA, et al. Sex differences in arterial stiffness and ventricular-arterial interactions. J Am Coll Cardiol 2013;61(1):96–103.
17. Segers P, Rietzschel ER, De Buyzere ML, et al. Noninvasive (input) impedance, pulse wave velocity, and wave reflection in healthy middle-aged men and women. Hypertension 2007;49(6):1248–55.
18. Waddell TK, Dart AM, Gatzka CD, et al. Women exhibit a greater age-related increase in proximal aortic stiffness than men. J Hypertens 2001;19(12):2205–12.
19. Schutte AE, Kruger R, Gafane-Matemane LF, et al. Ethnicity and arterial stiffness. Arterioscler Thromb Vasc Biol 2020;40(5):1044–54.
20. Brar I, Robertson AD, Hughson RL. Increased central arterial stiffness and altered cerebrovascular haemodynamic properties in South Asian older adults. J Hum Hypertens 2016;30(5):309–14.
21. Guo QH, Muhammad IF, Borné Y, et al. Difference in the risk profiles of carotid-femoral pulse wave velocity: results from two community-based studies in China and Sweden. J Hum Hypertens 2020;34(3):207–13.
22. Markert MS, Della-Morte D, Cabral D, et al. Ethnic differences in carotid artery diameter and stiffness: the Northern Manhattan Study. Atherosclerosis 2011; 219(2):827–32.

23. Park CM, Tillin T, March K, et al. Adverse effect of diabetes and hyperglycaemia on arterial stiffness in Europeans, South Asians, and African Caribbeans in the SABRE study. J Hypertens 2016;34(2):282–9.

24. Kaess BM, Rong J, Larson MG, et al. Aortic stiffness, blood pressure progression, and incident hypertension. JAMA 2012;308(9):875–81.

25. Domanski MJ, Davis BR, Pfeffer MA, et al. Isolated systolic hypertension. Hypertension 1999;34(3):375–80.

26. Loose S, Solou D, Strecker C, et al. Characterization of aortic aging using 3D multi-parametric MRI-long-term follow-up in a population study. Sci Rep 2023; 13(1):6285.

27. Chirinos JA, Segers P, Hughes T, et al. Large-artery stiffness in health and disease: JACC state-of-the-art review. J Am Coll Cardiol 2019;74(9):1237–63.

28. Chi C, Liu Y, Xu Y, et al. Association between arterial stiffness and heart failure with preserved ejection fraction. Front Cardiovasc Med 2021;8:707162.

29. Chow B, Rabkin SW. The relationship between arterial stiffness and heart failure with preserved ejection fraction: a systemic meta-analysis. Heart Fail Rev 2015; 20(3):291–303.

30. Feola M. The influence of arterial stiffness in heart failure: a clinical review. J Geriatr Cardiol 2021;18(2):135–40.

31. Wan J, Liu S, Yang Y, et al. Roles of arterial pressure volume index and arterial velocity pulse index trajectories in risk prediction in hypertensive patients with heart failure with preserved ejection fraction. Clin Exp Hypertens 2020;42(5): 469–78.

32. Mitchell GF. Arterial stiffness in aging: does it have a place in clinical practice? Hypertension 2021;77(3):768–80.

33. Weber T, O'Rourke MF, Ammer M, et al. Arterial stiffness and arterial wave reflections are associated with systolic and diastolic function in patients with normal ejection fraction. Am J Hypertens 2008;21(11):1194–202.

34. Safar ME, London GM, Plante GE. Arterial stiffness and kidney function. Hypertension 2004;43(2):163–8.

35. Zuo J, Hu Y, Chang G, et al. Relationship between arterial stiffness and chronic kidney disease in patients with primary hypertension. J Hum Hypertens 2020; 34(8):577–85.

36. Tian X, Chen S, Xia X, et al. Causal association of arterial stiffness with the risk of chronic kidney disease. JACC (J Am Coll Cardiol): Asia 2023. https://doi.org/10.1016/j.jacasi.2023.10.010.

37. Inserra F, Forcada P, Castellaro A, et al. Chronic kidney disease and arterial stiffness: a two-way path. Front Med (Lausanne) 2021;8:765924.

38. Elias MF, Robbins MA, Budge MM, et al. Arterial pulse wave velocity and cognition with advancing age. Hypertension 2009;53(4):668–73.

39. Waldstein SR, Rice SC, Thayer JF, et al. Pulse pressure and pulse wave velocity are related to cognitive decline in the Baltimore Longitudinal Study of Aging. Hypertension 2008;51(1):99–104.

40. Kearney-Schwartz A, Rossignol P, Bracard S, et al. Vascular structure and function is correlated to cognitive performance and white matter hyperintensities in older hypertensive patients with subjective memory complaints. Stroke 2009; 40(4):1229–36.

41. Hughes TM, Wagenknecht LE, Craft S, et al. Arterial stiffness and dementia pathology: atherosclerosis risk in communities (ARIC)-PET study. Neurology 2018; 90(14):e1248–56.

42. Tsao CW, Seshadri S, Beiser AS, et al. Relations of arterial stiffness and endothelial function to brain aging in the community. Neurology 2013;81(11):984–91.

43. Chirinos JA. Arterial stiffness: basic concepts and measurement techniques. Journal of cardiovascular translational research 2012;5:243–55.

44. O'Rourke M. Arterial stiffness, systolic blood pressure, and logical treatment of arterial hypertension. Hypertension 1990;15(4):339–47.

45. O'Rourke MF, Franklin SS. Arterial stiffness: reflections on the arterial pulse. Eur Heart J 2006;27(21):2497–8.

46. Lim MA, Townsend RR. Arterial compliance in the elderly: its effect on blood pressure measurement and cardiovascular outcomes. Clin Geriatr Med 2009;25(2):191–205.

47. Park S, Kwon M, Nam H, et al. Interpolation time-optimized aortic pulse wave velocity estimation by 4D flow MRI. Sci Rep 2023;13(1):16484.

48. Jarvis K, Scott MB, Soulat G, et al. Aortic pulse wave velocity evaluated by 4D flow MRI across the adult lifespan. J Magn Reson Imag 2022;56(2):464–73.

49. Harloff A, Mirzaee H, Lodemann T, et al. Determination of aortic stiffness using 4D flow cardiovascular magnetic resonance-a population-based study. J Cardiovasc Magn Reson 2018;20(1):43.

50. Asmar R, Benetos A, London G, et al. Aortic distensibility in normotensive, untreated and treated hypertensive patients. Blood Pres 1995;4(1):48–54.

51. O'Rourke MF, Pauca A, Jiang X-J. Pulse wave analysis. Br J Clin Pharmacol 2001;51(6):507.

52. Hajdusianek W, Żórawik A, Poręba R, et al. Assessment of aortic stiffness in computed tomography–methodology of radiological examination from 2000 to 2020. Pol J Radiol 2022;87:e635.

53. McEniery CM, McDonnell BJ, So A, et al. Aortic calcification is associated with aortic stiffness and isolated systolic hypertension in healthy individuals. Hypertension 2009;53(3):524–31.

54. Nowak KL, Rossman MJ, Chonchol M, et al. Strategies for achieving healthy vascular aging. Hypertension 2018;71(3):389–402.

55. Boutouyrie P, Lacolley P, Briet M, et al. Pharmacological modulation of arterial stiffness. Drugs 2011;71(13):1689–701.

56. Ong KT, Delerme S, Pannier B, et al. Aortic stiffness is reduced beyond blood pressure lowering by short-term and long-term antihypertensive treatment: a meta-analysis of individual data in 294 patients. J Hypertens 2011;29(6):1034–42.

57. Rey-Garcia J, Townsend RR. Large artery stiffness: a companion to the 2015 aha science statement on arterial stiffness. Pulse (Basel) 2021;9(1–2):1–10.

58. Laurent S, Boutouyrie P. Vascular Mechanism C. Dose-dependent arterial destiffening and inward remodeling after olmesartan in hypertensives with metabolic syndrome. Hypertension 2014;64(4):709–16.

59. Upala S, Wirunsawanya K, Jaruvongvanich V, et al. Effects of statin therapy on arterial stiffness: a systematic review and meta-analysis of randomized controlled trial. Int J Cardiol 2017;227:338–41.

60. Zhou YF, Wang Y, Wang G, et al. Association between statin use and progression of arterial stiffness among adults with high atherosclerotic risk. JAMA Netw Open 2022;5(6):e2218323.

61. Hickson LJ, Langhi Prata LGP, Bobart SA, et al. Senolytics decrease senescent cells in humans: preliminary report from a clinical trial of Dasatinib plus Quercetin in individuals with diabetic kidney disease. EBioMedicine 2019;47:446–56.

62. Justice JN, Nambiar AM, Tchkonia T, et al. Senolytics in idiopathic pulmonary fibrosis: results from a first-in-human, open-label, pilot study. EBioMedicine 2019;40:554–63.

63. Sugawara J, Tomoto T. Acute effects of short-term warm water immersion on arterial stiffness and central hemodynamics. Front Physiol 2021;12. https://doi.org/10.3389/fphys.2021.620201.

64. Li F, Liu J, Shan S, et al. Cold exposure attenuates medial arterial calcification via autophagy. Elsevier BV; 2023. https://www.researchgate.net/publication/369782953_Cold_Exposure_Attenuates_Medial_Arterial_Calcification_via_Autophagy.

65. Moreau K, Clayton Z, Dubose L, et al. Effects of regular exercise on vascular function with aging: does sex matter? Am J Physiol Heart Circ Physiol 2023. https://doi.org/10.1152/ajpheart.00392.2023.

66. Donato AJ, Eskurza I, Silver AE, et al. Direct evidence of endothelial oxidative stress with aging in humans. Circ Res 2007;100(11):1659–66.

67. Taddei S, Virdis A, Ghiadoni L, et al. Age-related reduction of NO availability and oxidative stress in humans. Hypertension 2001;38(2):274–9.

68. Stanek A, Grygiel-Górniak B, Brożyna-Tkaczyk K, et al. The influence of dietary interventions on arterial stiffness in overweight and obese subjects. Nutrients 2023/03;15(6). https://doi.org/10.3390/nu15061440.

69. Lichtenstein AH, Appel LJ, Vadiveloo M, et al. 2021 dietary guidance to improve cardiovascular health: a scientific statement from the american heart association. Circulation 2021;144(23). https://doi.org/10.1161/cir.0000000000001031.

70. D'Elia L, Galletti F, La Fata E, et al. Effect of dietary sodium restriction on arterial stiffness: systematic review and meta-analysis of the randomized controlled trials. J Hypertens 2018;36(4):734–43.

71. Masood W, Annamaraju P, Khan Suheb MZ, Uppaluri KR. Ketogenic Diet. 2023. In: StatPearls [Internet]. FL): StatPearls: Treasure Island; 2024.

72. Lange M, Coffey A, Coleman P, et al. Metabolic changes following intermittent fasting: a rapid review of systematic reviews. J Hum Nutr Diet 2023. https://doi.org/10.1111/jhn.13253.

73. Alinezhad-Namaghi M, Eslami S, Nematy M, et al. Association of time-restricted feeding, arterial age, and arterial stiffness in adults with metabolic syndrome. Health Science Reports 2023/07;6(7). https://doi.org/10.1002/hsr2.1385.

74. Coppola G, Natale F, Torino A, et al. The impact of the ketogenic diet on arterial morphology and endothelial function in children and young adults with epilepsy: a case–control study. Seizure 2014;23(4):260–5.

75. Arnett DK, Blumenthal RS, Albert MA, et al. 2019 ACC/AHA guideline on the primary prevention of cardiovascular disease: a report of the american college of cardiology/american heart association task force on clinical practice guidelines. Circulation 2019;140(11):e596–646.

76. Kim HC, Ihm SH, Kim GH, et al. 2018 Korean Society of Hypertension guidelines for the management of hypertension: part I-epidemiology of hypertension. Clin Hypertens 2019;25:16.

77. Umemura S, Arima H, Arima S, et al. The Japanese society of hypertension guidelines for the management of hypertension (JSH 2019). Hypertens Res 2019;42(9):1235–481.

78. Unger T, Borghi C, Charchar F, et al. 2020 International society of hypertension global hypertension practice guidelines. Hypertension 2020;75(6):1334–57.

General Principles, Etiologies, Evaluation, and Management in Older Adults

Brent M. Egan, MD[a,b,c,]*, Michael W. Rich, MD[d],
Susan E. Sutherland, PhD[a], Jackson T. Wright Jr, MD, PhD[e],
Sverre E. Kjeldsen, MD, PhD[f,g,1]

KEYWORDS

- Hypertension • Intensive treatment • Geriatrics • Cardiovascular risk factors
- Cardiovascular disease

KEY POINTS

- The benefits of intensive antihypertensive therapy outweigh the risks in older adults in the absence of dementia and severe frailty.
- Comprehensive initial assessment of cognitive and physical function is important in determining treatment intensity and identifying compelling indications for specific antihypertensive medication drug classes.
- In older adults with hypertension who are candidates for intensive antihypertensive therapy, both moderate sodium and weight reduction are successful lifestyle interventions to improve blood pressure (BP) control.
- The adage "start low and go slow" contributes to clinical inertia in managing BP among older adults.
- Assessment annually and following emergency department or hospital admission provide key opportunities to reassess patient proprities, treatment targets and indications or contraindication for specific antihypertensive medication classes.

[a] American Medical Association, 2 West Washington Street – Suite 601, Greenville, SC 29601, USA; [b] Medical University of South Carolina, Greenville, SC, USA; [c] Medical University of South Carolina, Charleston, SC, USA; [d] Washington University School of Medicine, 660 South Euclid Avenue, CB 8086, St Louis, MO 63110, USA; [e] Department of Medicine, College of Medicine, Case Western Reserve University, University Hospitals Case Medical Center, UH Cleveland Medical Center, 11100 Euclid Avenue, Cleveland, OH 44106, USA; [f] Department of Cardiology, University of Oslo, Institute of Clinical Medicine, Ullevaal Hospital, Kirkeveien 166, Oslo N-0407, Norway; [g] Department of Nephrology, University of Oslo, Institute of Clinical Medicine, Ullevaal Hospital, Kirkeveien 166, Oslo N-0407, Norway
[1] Present address: Sollerudveien 23D, N-0283 Oslo, Norway.
* Corresponding author. Medical University of South Carolina, 2 West Washington Street – Suite 601, Greenville, SC 29601.
E-mail address: brent.egan@ama-assn.org

Clin Geriatr Med 40 (2024) 551–571
https://doi.org/10.1016/j.cger.2024.04.008
0749-0690/24/© 2024 Elsevier Inc. All rights reserved.
geriatric.theclinics.com

INTRODUCTION

The prevalence of hypertension increases with age in all segments of the population. This article provides an overview of the etiology, pathophysiology, and general principles of evaluation and management of hypertension in older adults.

Blood pressure (BP) control over the lifespan promotes healthy aging: Elevated BP in mid-life is associated with cardiovascular disease (CVD) and dementia later in life.[1–3] Prevention and control of hypertension in middle adult years is important to healthy aging. Initiating and sustaining antihypertensive treatment in older adults is beneficial for reducing cardiovascular events and total mortality. The doubling of CVD risk per 20 mm Hg increment in systolic BP (SBP) is similar from the fifth through eighth decades. Absolute CVD risk doubles with each passing decade. While relative benefits of antihypertensive therapy are similar for adults in mid- and later life, absolute benefits are greater for older adults given higher absolute risk.[4,5] Hypertension as a cardiovascular risk factor continues in the ninth decade of life and beyond.[6]

Multiple chronic health conditions (CHCs) are common in older adults increasing from 18% at ages 18 to 44 years to 81% at ≥65 years.[7] Among Medicare beneficiaries with hypertension, 60% have 3 or more CHCs and only 5% have hypertension as an isolated condition.[8] The frequency of CHCs based on paid claims data is even higher when assessed from electronic health record data.[9] Common coexisting CHCs include hyperlipidemia, atherosclerotic CVD, cardiac arrhythmias, valvular heart disease, and heart failure, as well as osteoarthritis, obesity, behavioral health disorders, chronic lung disease, diabetes, hypothyroidism, fluid and electrolyte disorders, cancer, neurologic conditions including dementia, and chronic kidney disease.[7–9] Thus, integrated care is required to limit adverse outcomes, polypharmacy, and unnecessary health care utilization in older adults with hypertension.[9–11]

A comprehensive history, physical, and laboratory examination is important in older adults with hypertension given multisystem disease and behavioral health disorders. Thorough evaluation is required to determine BP targets, identify compelling indications for specific antihypertensive drugs classes, and avoid drug–drug and drug–disease interactions.[4,5,9]

Antihypertensive therapy and quality of life: Delaying and preventing CVD and dementia with effective antihypertensive therapy are compatible with high quality of life. While adverse events are reported more often in older than middle-aged adults with more intensive antihypertensive treatment, the absolute increase compared to standard treatment is similar.[4,5]

Previous recommendations to start low and go slow have limitations for many older adults: Among adults at high absolute CVD risk, events are reduced within the first 1 to 6 months of treatment with better BP control.[11–13] Monthly visits and therapeutic adjustments are appropriate for most older adults until hypertension is controlled.[4,5,14]

Frailty and cognitive impairment raise caution: More intensive antihypertensive therapy is beneficial in older adults with mild-to-moderate cognitive impairment and frailty. Benefits appear absent or reversed when significant cognitive impairment or advanced frailty is present.[4,5] Randomized clinical trials are needed to verify observational data in these high-risk populations.

Reassess annually and following intercurrent events: In older adults, annual evaluation and following changes in health status are appropriate for assessing conditions impacting treatment targets as well as compelling indications and contraindications for specific antihypertensive medication classes.[4,5]

Management should be individualized and patient-centered across the spectrum of older adults.[15,16] Shared decision-making including the patient and key individuals in the patient's life is essential, especially when cognitive impairment and frailty progress.

ETIOLOGIES

Age-related changes in the vasculature, sympathetic drive, and kidney function emerge as important factors underlying the progressive rise in prevalent hypertension with aging. In this section, office hypertension, masked hypertension, and pseudohypertension will also be addressed as these conditions disproportionately impact older adults.

Age-Related Vascular Changes

Vascular aging (stiffness) plays a major role in the age-related decline in diastolic blood pressure (DBP, mm Hg) and increases in SBP, pulse pressure, and prevalent hypertension.[5,17,18] SBP, pulse pressure, and prevalent hypertension rise more with age in women than men, which may reflect sex-related differences in vascular aging. Sympathetic drive rises more with age in women than men and may also contribute to greater age-related increases of SBP in women.[19] The greater age-related increase of SBP in Black than White adults may reflect racial differences in vascular aging possibly mediated by adverse social determinants of health.[20]

Age-Related Changes in Autonomic Function and Sympathetic Activity

Age-related increases in sympathetic drive contribute to the rise in prevalent hypertension with aging.[20] Autonomic dysfunction in older adults also contributes to age-related increases in orthostatic hypotension and supine hypertension. Consequently, BP should be measured in the standing position regularly in older adults 1 and 3 minutes after standing and after 10 minutes in selected patients, for example, syncope or falls that occur after a period of time in the upright position. A fall in SBP of $\geq$20 mm Hg or in DBP of $\geq$10 mm Hg within 3 minutes is associated with autonomic dysfunction and intensive diuretic and vasodilator therapy.[21–23] Orthostatic hypotension was reported in 4%, 7%, and 10% of patients in Systolic Hypertension in the Elderly Program,[24] Systolic Blood Pressure Intervention Trial (SPRINT),[25] and the Japanese[26] studies, respectively, and associated with adverse outcomes. Orthostatic hypertension, defined as $\geq$20 mm Hg rise of SBP on standing, was identified in one-fifth of adults (mean 83 years) referred to a geriatric center and was as common as orthostatic hypotension.[27] Orthostatic hypertension may point to masked hypertension.[28]

Damage to the afferent nerves, the brainstem, or the efferent limb of the baroreflex may result in various mild or severe BP abnormalities. Baroreflex failure may be caused by bilateral damage to carotid baroreceptors or baroreflex afferent nerves,[29–31] while damage to the efferent part of the baroreflex is often a component of other diseases.[31] Baroreflex failure is characterized by large BP variability with hypertensive surges, episodes of hypotension, and frequently orthostatic hypotension.[29–31] Because hypertensive episodes caused by baroreflex failure are mediated by uncontrolled sympathetic activation and worsened by physiologic and psychological stress, treatment with long-acting central sympatholytic agents may be effective.[32] Alcohol and smoking as well as diuretics and vasodilators can exacerbate orthostatic hypotension and should be avoided when possible. Severe hypotensive episodes are managed with fluid administration. Severe symptomatic bradycardia due to uncontrolled cardiac parasympathetic activation or sick sinus syndrome may prompt pacemaker implantation, although the BP response is variable.[33]

Autonomic failure is typically characterized by orthostatic hypotension frequently accompanied by supine hypertension.[34] It is essential to identify potentially treatable conditions, such as autoimmune-mediated autonomic ganglionopathies.[35] Symptomatic therapies such as lower limb venous compression and increased salt and water intake should first be tried.[36] Drugs that may worsen orthostatic hypotension should be discontinued when possible and include selective α_1-adrenoceptor antagonists (eg, doxazosin and prazosin), as well as relatively selective $\alpha1_{A/D}$ antagonists used to improve urine flow mainly in older men. In some cases, it is reasonable to combine α_1-adrenoceptor agonists and the selective antagonist of the alpha-1 subtype A receptor and alpha-1 subtype D receptor ($\alpha1_{A/D}$) antagonists to manage orthostatic hypotension, while limiting urine retention, analogous to using β_1-selective antagonists and β_2-selective agonists in patients with obstructive airways disease.

Pharmacologic treatment with α-adrenoreceptor agonists (eg, midodrine) or fludrocortisone to limit orthostasis can also exacerbate supine hypertension.[37] Supine hypertension typically increases urine excretion during the night, which worsens orthostatic hypotension the next day. Head-up tilt during sleep is recommended to reduce supine hypertension and nocturia and to reduce orthostasis the following day.[37] Antihypertensive therapies at bedtime can be considered in selected patients but need to be balanced against the risk for orthostatic hypotension and falls.[37]

White Coat Hypertension, Masked Hypertension, and Pseudohypertension

White coat hypertension (WCH) is defined by SBP in the clinical setting $\geq$10 mm Hg above values outside the clinic. The prevalence of WCH is estimated to be approximately 15% in the general population but up to 50% in older adults.[38] Recent studies indicate that WCH is associated with greater risk for cardiovascular events than nonhypertension but less than sustained hypertension.[38–40]

Masked hypertension occurs when the office BP is nonhypertensive but out-of-office BP is hypertensive.[41] The prevalence of masked hypertension is less well delineated, but it is associated with cardiovascular risk comparable to sustained hypertension in and out of office.[42] Both WCH and masked hypertension can be diagnosed by self-measured BP (SMBP) or 24 hour ambulatory BP monitoring (ABPM), although 24 hour ABPM is more sensitive than SMBP for detecting masked hypertension.[41] Treatment of WCH and masked hypertension is uncertain because to date there have been no clinical trials testing either lifestyle or pharmacologic interventions. While the 2017 American College of Cardiology / American Heart Association (ACC/AHA) hypertension guideline offers no specific therapeutic recommendations,[14] it is reasonable to treat patients with WCH or masked hypertension if hypertension-mediated organ damage is detected, for example, left ventricular hypertrophy (LVH) or chronic kidney disease.

Pseudohypertension refers to a condition where SBP or DBP measured noninvasively by cuff is greater than 10 mm Hg higher than intra-arterial values.[43] The condition is attributed to stiff noncompressible arteries and is especially common in older adults, with some series reporting up to 50% prevalence in select populations. However, most older adults with so-called pseudohypertension have true systolic hypertension and are at increased risk for end-organ damage, so the term is misleading and has fallen out of favor.

Age-Related Changes in Renal Function and Salt Sensitivity

Salt sensitivity of BP increases with age, coincident with age-related declines in renal blood flow and renal sodium excretion.[44,45] However, the link between age and salt sensitivity is more complex. Total renal blood flow is only weakly related to renal sodium excretion, whereas inner medullary flow, which is approximately 1% of overall renal blood flow, is strongly related to sodium excretion.[46] Moreover, the effects of drugs on renal medullary blood flow are much more closely associated with changes in renal tubular sodium excretion than changes in total renal blood flow. For example, renin–angiotensin system inhibitors induce sustained increases in renal medullary blood flow and lower BP without volume retention.[46]

Aging is also associated with increases in visceral fat and inflammation, even in the absence of weight gain or overt obesity.[47,48] Visceral fat and inflammation are associated with salt-sensitive hypertension.[49] Moderate sodium restriction lowers BP in relatively healthy older adults without major adverse effects.[50]

HISTORY, EXAMINATIONS, AND LABORATORY ASSESSMENT
General and Personal History

Key features include the history of hypertension, for example, age at hypertension diagnosis, history of BP values, and progression. Important aspects of the general, past medical, social and family histories, and review of systems are summarized in **Box 1**.[4] Historical features provide an assessment of the estimated duration and severity of hypertension, adherence to antihypertensive therapy, adverse effects and effectiveness as well as dietary patterns, potential target organ involvement, relevant comorbid conditions, and symptoms suggesting secondary hypertension, and relevant family history.

Physical Examination

In addition to a general physical examination, the examination is targeted at determining current BP values, target organ damage, and signs of secondary hypertension, as summarized in **Box 1**. Heart rate and BP are measured with standard protocols including orthostatic changes in BP and heart rate after 1 and 3 minutes standing.

Cardiovascular examination includes palpation and auscultation of the heart as well as auscultation of the lungs. In patients with LVH, the apical impulse is often sustained and may be laterally displaced. An fourth heart sound (S_4) gallop is often audible (in sinus rhythm) and may be palpable. An third heart sound (S_3) gallop generally indicates left ventricular systolic dysfunction and implies heart failure. Systolic murmurs due to aortic valve sclerosis/stenosis or mitral regurgitation are common but nonspecific. Lung examination may reveal wet crackles at the bases and above if heart failure is present but can be difficult to distinguish from atelectasis or chronic lung disease. The carotid and femoral arteries should be examined for bruits. Peripheral pulses should be checked in all extremities to assess for peripheral arterial disease.

The physical examination should include an assessment of physical frailty.[51] The Activities of Daily Living scale is another simple instrument for assessing physical function.[52] Various cognitive tests are available including the minimal mental status, Montreal Cognitive Assessment, and several other instruments.[53] Evaluation of physical and cognitive function is important in establishing a baseline, informing BP targets of antihypertensive therapy, and guiding an integrated care plan.

Standard laboratory testing is listed in **Box 1** and includes screening for target organ damage and commonly associated cardiovascular risk factors. Several equations are available for estimating glomerular filtration rate (eGFR) with relative advantages and disadvantages.[44,54,55] Given concerns raised, use of race-based equations has declined recently.

Box 1
Medical history, physical examination, and standard laboratory evaluation

Personal history
    Age at hypertension diagnosis, BP values, and rate of progression
    Current/past antihypertensive medications, effectiveness, adverse effects
    Adherence, reasons for limited adherence (cost, adverse effects, other)
    If female, previous hypertension in pregnancy, pre-eclampsia

Past medical, social, and family history
    Cigarette, tobacco history
    Dietary history (whole, processed foods), alcohol intake (frequency, amount)
    Physical activity (frequency, duration, intensity), sedentary time
    Weight history; maximum, minimum adult weight, weight cycling; weight loss medications,
    bariatric surgery
    History of sexual dysfunction
    Sleep history, latency, duration, early awakening, snoring, sleep apnea (history from partner)
    Frequency, intensity, duration of life stresses
    History of other chronic diseases (neurologic, cancer, liver/digestive, musculoskeletal, skin)
    Family history of hypertension, diabetes, CVD, stroke, kidney disease

Review of systems, symptoms of target organ damage
    Neurologic: headache, vertigo, syncope, impaired vision, transient ischemic attack (TIA),
    sensory or motor deficit, stroke, carotid revascularization, cognitive impairment, memory
    loss, dementia/cognitive impairment (refer to tests)
    Heart: chest pain, dyspnea (rest, activity, position), edema, myocardial infarction, coronary
    revascularization, syncope, palpitations, arrhythmias (especially atrial fibrillation [AF]), heart
    failure
    Kidney: thirst, polyuria, nocturia, hesitancy, decreased stream, hematuria, urinary tract
    infections
    Peripheral arteries: cold extremities, intermittent claudication, pain-free walking distance,
    pain at rest, ulcer or necrosis, peripheral revascularization

History suggesting possible secondary hypertension
    Onset of hypertension less than 40 years especially with BP $\geq$150/$\geq$95, sudden development
    or rapid worsening
    History of recurrent renal/urinary tract disease, infection
    Repetitive sweating, headache, anxiety, palpitations (possible pheochromocytoma)
    History spontaneous or diuretic-provoked hypokalemia, episodic muscle weakness
    (hyperaldosteronism)
    History, heat intolerance, weight loss (hyperthyroidism); weakness, kidney stones
    (hyperparathyroidism)
    Women: reproductive history, contraceptive or hormone use, postmenopausal status
    Drugs (other than antihypertensive) include nonprescription drugs and supplements

Physical examination vital signs
    Weight and height, calculate body mass index (BMI)
    Waist circumference
    BP and heart rate seated (2–3 measurements; preferably automated office BP)
    BP and heart rate after 1 and 3 minutes standing
    Signs of hypertension-mediated organ damage
    Neurologic examination and cognitive status
    Fundoscopic examination for hypertensive retinopathy, retinal vascular change
    Palpation and auscultation of heart (enlargement, extra sounds, murmurs) carotid arteries
    (pulses, bruits)
    Palpation and auscultation of abdominal aorta, femoral arteries (aneurysm, bruits)
    Ankle brachial index
    Signs of secondary hypertension
    Skin: cafe-au-lait patches of neurofibromatosis (pheochromocytoma)
    Abdominal palpation for signs of renal enlargement (polycystic kidneys)
    Auscultation renal arteries (bruits)

Moon face, abdominal obesity, striae, telangiectasia, bruising, female hirsutism, fat pads (collarbone, back of neck), hyperpigmentation (Cushing's); frontal bossing, overgrowth jaw, nose, ears (acromegaly)

Tachycardia, atrial arrhythmia, moist skin, fine tremor (hyperthyroidism)

Selected standard laboratory tests for workup of hypertensive patients

Hemoglobin and/or hematocrit

Fasting blood glucose and glycosylated hemoglobin (HbA1c)

Blood lipids: total cholesterol, high-density lipoprotein (HDL) cholesterol, triglycerides, low-density lipoprotein cholesterol (LDL), non-HDL

Blood sodium, potassium, chloride, and CO2 (bicarbonate)

Serum creatine (cystatin C) for estimating glomerular filtration rate (eGFR)

Blood calcium, albumin, uric acid

Urine analysis (preferably first voided urine in the morning), multicomponent dipstick, albumin/creatinine ratio

A 12 lead ECG

Ankle brachial index if diminished pedal pulses or symptoms of claudication

From: Mancia G, Kreutz R, Brunström M, Burnier M, Grassi G, Januszewicz A, Muiesan ML, Tsioufis K, Agabiti-Rosei E, et al. 2023 ESH Guidelines for the management of arterial hypertension. J Hypertension 2023;41:1874-2071.

Other Artery, Heart, Kidney, or Brain Examinations

A 24 hour ABPM may be useful in older patients to confirm a diagnosis of hypertension, verify adequacy of BP control, detect low BP in patients who suffer from dizziness and/or postprandial or orthostatic hypotension and investigate nighttime BP and hypertension (an indication for giving at least some of the BP medication at bedtime in nondippers or reverse dippers). SMBP or home BP provides similar prognostic information as 24 hour ABPM but may be less accurate, especially for detecting masked hypertension, and does not include nighttime measurements.

Echocardiography can provide important diagnostic and prognostic information but is not routinely recommended absent indications from the history, physical, and standard laboratory evaluation. Common findings in older adults include LVH, left atrial enlargement, and evidence for diastolic dysfunction. LVH may regress when BP is well controlled; regression is prognostically beneficial. Previous myocardial infarction (wall motion abnormalities) and valvular defects such as aortic stenosis and mitral regurgitation may be detected (and explain systolic murmur by auscultation).

Ultrasound examinations of the kidneys, aorta, and carotid arteries may be indicated based on the history, physical, and laboratory examination. Doppler studies of renal arteries to assess for renal artery stenosis and CT or MRI scans of various organs including the brain may provide needed information but are not routinely recommended for evaluation of hypertension in the absence of specific indications. Large arteries may be assessed by ankle–brachial index, pulse wave velocity, and other tests to verify arterial stiffness.

More extensive testing may clarify the presence and severity of hypertension-mediated organ damage, which can impact treatment targets and constitute compelling indications for specific classes of antihypertensive medications.

COMMON CAUSES OF SECONDARY HYPERTENSION
Sleep Apnea

Sleep disturbances may contribute to high BP. Both obstructive sleep apnea[56] and central sleep apnea,[57] which is associated with stroke, heart failure, and narcotic use, are relatively common in older adults with hypertension. Recurrent hypoxia strongly activates the sympathetic nervous system and causes nighttime hypertension without dipping. Sustained BP elevation during the day can occur. Patients are frequently obese. Weight reduction reduces the severity of sleep apnea and is strongly recommended for older adults who are weight loss candidates (see lifestyle interventions, weight loss). Patients can be screened for obstructive sleep apnea using one of the validated questionnaires.[58] Effective treatment with continuous positive airway pressure can have multiple beneficial effects including BP reduction, though less in older than younger patients. Surgery may be considered for individuals with severe sleep apnea who cannot tolerate or do not respond to more conservative interventions. All major antihypertensive drug classes can be used as needed to control BP.

Renal Artery Stenosis

Fibromuscular dysplasia, mostly in young to middle-aged women, and arteriosclerotic plaques, primarily in older patients, can cause critical renal artery stenosis and hypertension including apparent treatment-resistant hypertension.[4,14,59,60] Randomized trials of medical versus surgical management of patients with presumed renal artery hypertension have not produced consistent results, largely due to methodological limitations. Most specialists currently recommend invasive catheter-based treatment with or without stenting for stenoses ≥80%. Hypertension in older patients with atherosclerotic renovascular hypertension is typically treated medically including after anatomically successful revascularization, since hypertension is rarely cured in this group. Preservation of kidney function in patients with significant bilateral or unilateral stenosis and a solitary kidney has been more successful with revascularization. Medical therapy of renal artery stenosis, both unilateral and bilateral, includes an angiotensin converting enzyme (ACE) inhibitor or angiotensin receptor blocker (ARB; renin-angiotensin system [RAS] blocker), calcium channel blockers, and diuretics when necessary. Careful monitoring of eGFR is important in patients with renovascular hypertension as BP reduction alone may acutely lower renal blood flow and decrease eGFR. In addition to lowering BP, RAS blockers dilate the postglomerular efferent arteriole, which can reduce filtration fraction and eGFR. Volume depletion in patients with renovascular hypertension further activates the RAS system and the likelihood of large reductions in eGFR with RAS blocker therapy. Yet, most patients, even with bilateral renal artery disease or unilateral disease and a solitary kidney, will not have ≥30% reductions in eGFR during RAS blocker therapy.[60,61]

Primary Aldosteronism

Primary aldosteronism, described initially in 1955,[62] is common, detected in up to 20% of middle-aged and older patients with more severe or apparent treatment-resistant hypertension. With greater screening for primary aldosteronism, bilateral hyperplasia (60%–70%) is more common than unilateral aldosterone-producing adenoma (APA).[60] Hypokalemia is common with unilateral APA but less common with bilateral adrenal hyperplasia. Screening tests include documenting high aldosterone values in a plasma sample or a 24 hour urine collection in the presence of suppressed plasma renin activity. In primary aldosteronism, the aldosterone–renin ratio is typically greater than 30 but this also occurs in low-renin hypertension without excess aldosterone. While plasma aldosterone is simpler to obtain, a 24 hour urine collection is a better screening test for excess aldosterone production. Nonsuppressibility of aldosterone with a high-sodium diet or normal saline infusion confirms the diagnosis of primary aldosteronism. Treatment includes laparoscopic removal of APA and medical therapy with mineralocorticoid antagonists for bilateral hyperplasia. Selective adrenal vein sampling for aldosterone is recommended before unilateral adrenalectomy as incidental nonfunctioning adenomas are relatively common. The dosing of mineralo-corticoid receptor antagonists is determined in part by an increase in plasma renin activity to a ratio greater than 1 as a marker that aldosterone is sufficiently blocked.

MANAGEMENT

Management is directed at controlling BP to target, minimizing cardiovascular events, and maintaining cognitive function,[4,14,63] while limiting adverse effects and maintaining quality of life. Target BP is informed by prior clinical trials (Supiano MA),[64] which are summarized briefly later.

Treatment Targets

Multiple randomized controlled trials (RCTs) and meta-analyses document that antihypertensive therapy reduces cardiovascular morbidity and mortality and all-cause mortality in older adults with systolic/diastolic or isolated systolic hypertension (**Table 1**[64–79]). Although most trials excluded adults aged 80 years or more, HYVET focused exclusively on this age group.[76] SPRINT enrolled 2636 patients ≥75 years of age (mean 79.9 years, 38% women), including patients with mild–moderate frailty and slow gait speed. Similar benefit was noted in SPRINT participants ≥80 year old.[79] In addition, benefit was demonstrated for intensive treatment even among those in the lowest DBP quintile at baseline (61±5 mm Hg), which disputes the J curve concern.[80]

The STEP trial[79] showed that treatment to SBP target of 110 to 129 (mean 126.7) in hypertensive people aged 60 to 80 years resulted in a lower incidence of cardiovascular complications than standard treatment with an SBP target of 130 to 149 (mean 135.9). Cardiovascular benefit was also documented among older SPRINT patients who achieved a mean on-treatment SBP of 123.4 with intensive versus 134.8 with standard treatment.[77] Given current evidence, targeting BP less than 120/70 is not recommended,[4] although many older adults will have DBP less than 70 when SBP targets are attained.[70]

Since the benefits of treatment include striking reductions in stroke (mean 32%) and heart failure (mean 48%), it is highly likely that quality of life, functional capacity, and maintenance of independence are all enhanced with antihypertensive therapy. In addition, there is a growing body of evidence that treatment of hypertension is associated with a modest but significant reduction in incident dementia and cognitive decline, as reviewed in de Havenon and colleagues' study.[80]

Lifestyle interventions

Sodium restriction. Salt sensitivity is associated with age-related increases of BP, and salt sensitivity increases with age.[45,81] The randomized Trial of Nonpharmacologic Intervention in the Elderly (TONE) included 975 independent adults 60 to 80 years without major physical or mental illness.[50] At baseline, participants had BP less than 145/85 mm Hg on antihypertensive monotherapy or single-pill combination (SPC) including a diuretic and nondiuretic drug class. In TONE, a 40 mmol/d reduction in sodium, from approximately 3.5 (which is common in the United States) to 2.5 g daily, lowered BP by 4/2 mm Hg. The primary outcome of SBP ≥150 mm Hg, DBP ≥90 over 3 visits of medication (stopped at month 3), restarting antihypertensive medication, or a cardiovascular event was reduced by 31% among adults randomized to reduced sodium. The primary outcome also occurred significantly less often in adults of African descent. Given limited data and the potential for unintended reductions of nutrient intake for adults aged 80 years or greater, the 2023 European Society of Hypertension (ESH) guideline does

Table 1
Clinical trials of hypertension in older adults

						Risk Reduction, %				
Trial	Year	N	Age	Entry BP	BP Difference	CVA	CAD	HF	CVD
HDFP	1976	2374	60–69	DBP ≥90; SC 101.6; RC 100.9	DBP –5.3 SC vs RC year 2	44	15	NR	16
ANBP-1	1981	582	60–69	DBP 95–109; SBP <200	DBP –6.3 Rx vs P	33	18	NR	31
EWPHE	1985	840	>60	SBP 160–239 and DBP 90–119	–23/–9 Rx vs P year 3	36	20	22	29
Coope	1986	884	60–79	SBP ≥170 or DBP ≥105	–18/–11 Rx vs control	42	–3	32	24
STOP-HTN	1991	1627	70–84	180–230/≥90 or <180/105–120	–19.5/–8.1 Rx vs P	47	13	51	40
SHEP	1991	4736	≥60	≥160/<90	–12/–4 Rx vs P	33	27	55	32
MRC	1992	4396	65–74	160–209/<115	a –15/–7 Rx vs P	25	19	NR	17
STONE	1996	1632	60–79	SBP 160–219 or DBP 90–124	–9.3/–5.6 Rx vs P	57	6	68	60
Syst-Eur	1997	4695	≥60	160–219/<95	SBP –10.5 Rx vs P	42	26	36	31
Syst-China	2001	2394	≥60	160–219/<95	–9.1/–3.2 Rx vs P	38	33	38	37
bANBP-2	2003	6083	65–84	SBP ≥160 or BP ≥140/90	–26/–12 diuretic and ACEI	12	14	15	11
HYVET	2008	3845	≥80	160–199/<110	–15/–6 Rx vs P	30	28	64	34
SPRINT	2016	2636	≥75	SBP 130–180, mean 141.6	–11.4/–5.2 intensive vs standard	28	31	38	34
STEP	2021	8511	60–80	140–189/≥60 or Rx	SBP –9.2 intensive vs standard	33	33	73	26
Weighted average						32.2	23.4	48.0	27.3

Trials and Reports that Included Adults <60 and ≥60 y

Trial	Year	N	Age	Entry BP	BP Difference	Risk Reduction, %			
						CVA	CAD	HF	CVD
ACCORD	2010	4733	≥40	Mean 139/76	SBP −14.2 intensive vs standard	47	6	6	12
SPRINT	2015	9361	≥50	Mean 140/78	SBP −14.8 intensive vs standard	11	12	33	25
RESPECT	2019	1263	50–85	130–180/80–110	−6.5/−3.3 intensive vs standard	27	NR	NR	NR
ESPRIT	2023	11,255	≥50			12	NR	NR	12
Weighted average						*18.6*	*10.0*	*23.9*	*16.8*

Abbreviations: ANBP-1, Australian National Blood Pressure, study 1; ANBP-2, Australian National Blood Pressure, study 2; Coope, Coope and Warrender; CAD, coronary artery disease; CVA, cerebrovascular accident; DBP, diastolic BP; EWPHE, European Working Party on Hypertension in the Elderly; HDFP, hypertension detection and follow-up program; HF, heart failure; HYVET, hypertension in the very elderly trial; MRC, Medical Research Council; NR, not reported; P, placebo; RC, referred care; RESPECT, recurrent stroke prevention clinical outcome study; Rx, pharmacotherapy; SBP, systolic BP; SC, stepped care; SHEP, Systolic Hypertension in the Elderly Program; SPRINT, Systolic Blood Pressure Intervention Trial; STEP, Strategy of Blood Pressure Intervention in the Elderly Hypertensive Patients; STONE, Shanghai Trial of Nifedipine in the Elderly; STOP-HTN, Swedish Trial of Older Patients with Hypertension; Syst-China, Systolic hypertension in China study; Syst-Eur, Systolic hypertension in Europe study.

[a] Estimated from figure.

[b] Diuretic versus ACEI.

not recommend salt restriction for adults in this age group unless daily consumption exceeds 10 g (~4 g sodium).[4]

While there are many healthy eating plans available, two of the most widely studied include the Dietary Approaches to Stop Hypertension (DASH) eating plan and the Mediterranean diet.

Dietary approaches to stop hypertension eating plan. The original report on the DASH eating plan included adults 22 years and older (mean 44 years). In a subset of 72 individuals with isolated systolic hypertension (mean age ~54 years), DASH lowered SBP 11.2 mm Hg, whereas the fruits and vegetables diet lowered SBP 8.1 mm Hg.[82] A systematic review and meta-analysis reported that DASH was still effective but significantly less so for lowering SBP and DBP in adults aged 50 years or greater than below 50 years.[83]

Mediterranean-style diet, which is moderate in sodium, lowered SBP by 5.5 mm Hg and decreased arterial stiffness in adults 65 to 79 year old.[84] The Mediterranean diet is associated with longevity[85] and likely beneficial to octogenarians as well.

Weight loss. Among obese adults in TONE (n = 585, age 60–80 years), the primary composite outcome of a hypertension diagnosis, requirement for beginning or restarting antihypertensive medications or cardiovascular event during up to 3 years of follow-up was reduced 36% with approximately 4 kg weight loss, 40% with sodium restriction, and 53% for weight loss and sodium restriction combined.[50] The investigators concluded that reducing sodium intake and weight were feasible, effective, and safe interventions for older persons with hypertension, recognizing participants were healthy. Caution has been raised about weight loss in older adults, although combining weight loss with aerobic and resistance training in older adults appears to maintain muscle mass and strength.[86] However, data in adults aged 80 years or greater are limited, which raises caution on weight loss intervention in this age group unless robust and markedly obese,[4] although the ACC/AHA guideline did not raise concerns.[14]

Physical activity. A systematic review and meta-analysis in adults aged 60 years or more reported that aerobic and resistance physical activity lowered BP by approximately 5.7/3.7 mm Hg.[87] Moderate- and high-intensity aerobic exercise are recommended for BP reduction,[14] but may not be possible or preferred by many older adults. Low-intensity physical activity for 6 minutes hourly reduced SBP greater than 10 mm Hg in overweight and obese highly sedentary adults (mean age 62 years).[88] Other data suggest that low-intensity physical activity is as effective as moderate- and high-intensity physical activity for diabetes prevention.[89]

Antihypertensive therapy: attaining benefit while limiting risk and adverse events

Pharmacotherapy for hypertension in older patients should aim to achieve the BP targets[4,14,64,90,91,92] while limiting adverse effects. In this regard, it is important to remember that intensive therapy when indicated is not associated with a lower probability that BP will fall ≥20/10 mm Hg with standing and injurious falls do not increase significantly.[77] In older patients and particularly those with mild–moderate frailty, initial antihypertensive monotherapy may be considered the first treatment step for baseline SBP 140 to 159. Since controlling systolic hypertension in older adults may be difficult, even in adults with untreated SBP 140 to 159, physicians should consider an initial 2 drug combination in most fit patients, beginning with low doses, for example, one-half standard or one-quarter maximum recommended, then up-titrating both doses and adding a third drug when needed to control SBP.

Initial combination treatment with half standard-to-standard doses of 2 antihypertensive drug classes in an SPC is recommended for most older patients with initial SBP 160 or greater.[4,14] SPCs are associated with better adherence and BP control as well as fewer cardiovascular events.[93] Better adherence to antihypertensive therapy is associated with fewer major adverse cardiovascular events, even in frail older adults.[4] More than half of older patients are exposed to polypharmacy due to multiple chronic conditions,[94] so limiting pill count and unnecessary medications is important.

HYVET and SPRINT showed that treating hypertension in adults aged 80 years or more including those with mild–moderate frailty reduced cardiovascular events.[95,96] Thus, antihypertensive drug treatment should be prescribed in most very old hypertensive patients, including those with mild-to-moderate frailty.

No RCT data are available in patients ≥90 years. Data on therapeutic strategies and BP targets are also missing in patients who reside in long-term care facilities or those with severe loss of autonomy, since virtually all trials in older adults excluded these individuals as well as those with limited life expectancy.[65–79] Several observational studies in older adults with severe frailty reported that morbidity and mortality are higher at lower BP values.[97,98] While such observations may be influenced by residual confounding and reflect selection bias, assessment of frailty status is recommended and currently impacts treatment targets as noted in this review.

Class-specific drug algorithms with attention to compelling indications

For older adults, any of the 4 major drug classes with documented benefit on morbidity and mortality in RCTs can be used (ACE inhibitor or ARB, calcium channel blocker [CCB], diuretic).[4,14] Older patients are more susceptible to adverse effects from β-blockers, such as fatigue or sleep-related disorders,[99] and can have a lesser antihypertensive response than the 4 classes listed as initial therapy. Therefore, beta-blockers should not be initial therapy in older adults in the absence of compelling indications.[4,14] In clinical practice, there are several common conditions in older adults for which beta-blockers are indicated, including heart failure and coronary heart disease.[4,14]

The treatment algorithm in **Table 2** represents one recommended sequence for older adults absent compelling indications for specific BP medication classes. For fit older patients, initial standard doses (half recommended maximum dose) are reasonable. As frailty increases, half standard doses are prudent, especially when starting treatment with an SPC. Following the treatment algorithm with the recommended monthly follow-up when BP is uncontrolled leads to a high probability of

Table 2
One antihypertensive treatment algorithm absent compelling indications

Rx Step	Initial Combination Rx	Initial Monotherapy
1	CCB + RASB (1/2 std to std doses)	CCB (std dose)
2	Double doses CCB and RASB	Add RASB (std dose); preferably Step 1 + 2SPC
3	Add TTD (prefer SPC; 3 meds, 1 pill)	Add TTD (std dose): prefer SPC (3 meds, 1 pill)
4	Maximum doses if std doses tolerated	Maximum doses if std doses tolerated
5	Add MRA or β-blocker at ½ std dose	Add MRA or β-blocker at ½ std dose

Abbreviations: CCB, calcium channel blocker; MRA, mineralocorticoid antagonist (eGFR >50, serum K+ <4.5); β-blocker, beta-adrenergic receptor blocker; RASB, renin–angiotensin system blocker, that is, ACEI, angiotensin-converting enzyme inhibitor or ARB, angiotensin receptor blocker; Rx, pharmacotherapy; SPC, single-pill combination; std, standard dose which is generally ½ maximum recommended; TTD, thiazide-type diuretic.

controlled BP within 6 months of initiating therapy (or earlier), which is associated with better cardiovascular outcomes. Good clinical judgment is needed to balance benefit and risk for individual patients, especially with more severe frailty.

Sodium-glucose cotransport type 2 (SGLT2) inhibitors, while not listed as antihypertensive agents, have natriuretic and sympatholytic properties.[100] SGLT2 inhibitors lower SBP by 4 to 8 mm Hg in adults with diabetes and hypertension,[101,102] a group with sympathetic activation and salt-sensitive hypertension.[103] SGLT2 inhibitors are not indicated for treating hypertension, but many older adults have diabetes, heart failure, or chronic kidney disease for which SGLT2 inhibitors are indicated. SGLT2 inhibitors lower BP among individuals with heart failure or chronic kidney disease.[104,105]

Management of apparent treatment-resistant hypertension

This topic is addressed in Vongpatanasin, Giacona[106] and briefly here. Patients with BP above goal on three or more antihypertensive drug classes have apparent treatment-resistant hypertension until common contributors to pseudoresistance are excluded: (1) nonhypertensive BP outside the clinic; (2) inadequate antihypertensive regimen prescribed (should include ≥3 antihypertensive medications at maximal or maximally tolerated doses); and (3) suboptimal adherence. In addition, it is important to identify and address key lifestyle factors such as high salt or alcohol intake.[59]

A small proportion of patients with apparent resistance have true treatment-resistant hypertension. After excluding pseudoresistance, identify and stop or minimize supplements and medications which raise BP. Evaluation for secondary causes of hypertension is important, especially when the preceding steps fail to control BP.[4,14,59,106] If uncontrolled BP persists after additionally excluding or addressing secondary causes, then adding a fourth drug is reasonable. In general, the US guidelines[14] recommend mineralocorticoid antagonists more strongly than other drugs as fourth-line agents, when eGFR is greater than 50 mL/min/1.73 m^2 and serum potassium (K$^+$) less than 4.6 meq/L, whereas the ESH guidelines[4] recommend beta-blockers. Monthly follow-up with review of current BP, medications, and adherence as well as further therapeutic adjustment is important until BP is controlled or best achievable BP obtained.

Device-based therapies can be considered in older adults with resistant hypertension. Renal denervation lowers ambulatory BP similarly to a single antihypertensive drug.[107,108] Age is not a significant factor in the BP response to renal denervation,[105] but the procedure lowers SBP less in patients with Isolated Systolic Hypertension (ISH) than those with combined systolic/diastolic hypertension.[108] Baroreceptor stimulation[109] is approved for heart failure in the United States and for heart failure and hypertension in Europe.

Long-Term Follow-up and Monitoring

General considerations

Chronologic aging is constant, whereas physiologic aging is variable. Even within individuals, physiologic aging is often nonlinear. Comorbid chronic conditions increase sharply with advancing age and include frailty, cognitive impairment, and dementia. Thus, comprehensive annual assessment is appropriate. More frequent evaluation is warranted when major events occur, often associated with hospital or emergency department admissions which are sometimes due to adverse drug effects. A patient-centered and engaged approach is essential not only during the initial evaluation and selection of target BP but also in revising target BP and care plans as appropriate for significant changes in health status.

Blood pressure and cardiovascular status

Long-term monitoring of BP, including out-of-office BP, is important in older patients. Orthostatic hypotension is common in adults greater than 65 years, even in the absence of symptoms, and associated with increased risk for falls. Consequently, routinely assessing BP taken after 1 and 3 minutes of standing is strongly recommended. Orthostasis after 6 minutes standing was also associated with risk of falls.[110] Patients or family members may be trained to perform home BP monitoring to determine average out-of-office BP and the range of BP given greater SBP variability in older than in middle-aged and younger adults.

Home BP taken by family members is recommended in patients with dementia, neurocognitive conditions, or physical limitations. A 24 hour ABPM is recommended in older patients with unresolved questions on the severity of hypertension, episodes of hypotension, or adequacy of control. In patients with dizziness, which is the most common adverse effect of antihypertensive treatment in older adults, ABPM may identify sustained hypotension or hypotensive episodes, for example, postprandial hypotension. In some older patients, ABPM may provide prognostically important information with therapeutic implications. For example, while taking antihypertensive drugs in the morning is recommended, nondipping and reverse dipping status are associated with greater cardiovascular risk. In this setting, nighttime dosing of at least one antihypertensive medication is reasonable. In less frequent cases with excessive nighttime dipping, avoiding bedtime dosing is appropriate given risk for ischemic events with nocturnal hypotension.

Assessing frailty and mental status is recommended prior to initiating antihypertensive treatment in older patients and annually to monitor changes in status, which impact treatment targets. Progressive deprescribing may be considered in patients with seated SBP less than 120 mm Hg, clinically significant orthostatic hypotension,[110–112] or who progress to severe frailty in whom strict control may be detrimental. The BP targets in adults with severe frailty and dementia are based on observational data and may be modified pending results of ongoing RCTs.

CLINICS CARE POINTS

- Healthy aging includes good BP control earlier in life.

- Shared decision making when selecting treatment goals and developing a treatment plan is important in respecting patient autonomy and engaging the patient (and caregivers) in effective self-management.

- Older adults without severe frailty or significant cognitive impairment, benefit from strict blood pressure control (mean systolic BP <130 mmHg).

- Aim to control hypertension in the first six months of management with monthly follow-up and treatment intensifications when BP is uncontrolled.

- Out-of-office BP monitoring in older adults can help in detecting post-prandial hypotension, assessing orthostatic symptoms, and office BP effects, which are all more common in older than younger adults.

DISCLOSURE

B.M. Egan received royalties (UpToDate) and a consultant with Mineralys (no honorarium or travel expenses). S.E. Kjeldsen received lecture honoraria from Emcure, Getz, J.B. Pharma, Merck Healthcare KGaA, and Vector-Intas.

REFERENCES

1. Liu M, Zhang S, Chen X, et al. Association of mid- to late-life blood pressure patterns with risk of subsequent coronary heart disease .and death. Front Cardiovasc Med 2021;8:632514.
2. Ou Y-N, Tan CC, Shen X-N, et al. Blood pressure and risks of cognitive impairment and dementia: a systematic review and meta-analysis of 209 prospective studies. Hypertension 2020;76:217–25.
3. Cohen LP, Vittinghoff E, Pletcher MJ, et al. Association of midlife cardiovascular risk factors with risk of heart failure subtypes later in life. J Cardiac Fail 2021;27: 435–44.
4. Mancia G, Kreutz R, Brunström M, et al. 2023 ESH Guidelines for the management of arterial hypertension. J Hypertension 2023;41:1874–2071.
5. Egan BM, Mattix-Kramer HJ, Basile JN, et al. Managing hypertension in older adults. Curr Hypertension Rep 2023;26:157–67.
6. Stokes JIII, Kannel WB, Wolf PA, et al. Blood pressure as a risk factor for cardiovascular disease. Hypertension 1989;13(Suppl 1):I13–9.
7. Buttorff C, Ruder T, Bauman M. Multiple chronic conditions in the United States. Santa Monica (CA): RAND Corporation; 2017.
8. Centers for Medicare and Medicaid Services. Chronic Conditions among Medicare Beneficiaries, Chartbook, 2012 Edition. Baltimore, MD. 2012.
9. Egan BM, Sutherland SE, Tilkemeier PL, et al. A cluster-based approach for integrating clinical management of Medicare beneficiaries with multiple chronic conditions. PLoS One 2019;14(6):e0217696.
10. Institute of Medicine Committee on Quality of Health Care in America. Crossing the quality chasm: a new health system for the 21st century. National Academy Press; 2001.
11. Weber MA, Julius S, Kjeldsen SE, et al. Blood pressure dependent and independent effects of antihypertensive treatment on clinical events in the VALUE Trial. Lancet 2004;363:2049–51.
12. Mariampillai JE, Eskås PA, Heimark S, et al. A case for less intensive blood pressure control: it matters to achieve target blood pressure early and sustained below 140/90 mmHg. Prog Cardiovasc Dis 2016;59:209–18.
13. Egan BM. Editorial commentary: prognostic value of blood pressure control delay in newly diagnosed hypertensive patients. J Hypertension 2019;37:290–1.
14. Whelton PK, Carey RM, Aronow WS, et al. 2017 ACC/AHA Guideline for the prevention, detection, evaluation, and management of high blood pressure in adults. Hypertension 2018;71:e13–115.
15. Shepherd J, Gurney S, Patel HP. Shared decision making and personalised care support planning: pillars of integrated care for older people. Clin Integrated Care 2022;12:100097.
16. Brown EL, Poltawski L, Pitchforth E, et al. Shared decision making between older people with multimorbidity and GPs: a qualitative study. Br J Gen Prac 2022;72:e609–18.
17. Tuday E, et al. The role of vascular aging in the development of hypertension. Clin Geriatr Med 2024;40(4).
18. Osude N, Durzao-Arvizu R, Markossian T, et al. Age and sex disparities in hypertension control: the multi-ethnic study of atherosclerosis (MESA). Am J Prev Cardiol 2021;8:100230.
19. Klassen SA, Joyner MJ, Baker SE. The impact of ageing and sex on sympathetic neurocirculatory regulation. Semin Cell Dev Biol 2021;116:72–81.

20. Reges O, Krefman AE, Hardy ST, et al. Race- and sex-specific factors associated with age-related slopes in systolic blood pressure: findings from the CARDIA Study. Hypertension 2023;80:1890–9.
21. Dani M, Dirksen A, Taraborrelli P, et al. Orthostatic hypotension in older people: considerations, diagnosis and management. Clin Med 2021;21:e275–82.
22. Freeman R, Wieling W, Axelrod FB, et al. Consensus statement on the definition of orthostatic hypotension, neurally mediated syncope and the postural tachycardia syndrome. Clin Auton Res 2011;21:69–72.
23. Jordan J, Ricci F, Hoffmann F, et al. Orthostatic hypertension: critical appraisal of an overlooked condition. Hypertension 2020;75:1151–8.
24. Kostis WJ, Sargsyan D, Mekkaoui C, et al. Association of orthostatic hypertension with mortality in the systolic hypertension in the elderly program. J Hum Hypertens 2019;33:735–40.
25. Rahman M, Pradhan N, Chen Z, et al. Orthostatic hypertension and intensive blood pressure control; post-Hoc analyses of SPRINT. Hypertension 2021;77:49–58.
26. Hoshide S, Matsui Y, Shibasaki S, et al. Orthostatic hypertension detected by self-measured home blood pressure monitoring: a new cardiovascular risk factor for elderly hypertensives. Hypertens Res 2008;31:1509–16.
27. Rosa F, Rougette K, Zmude L, et al. Association bewween orthostatis blood pressure dysregulation and geriatiric syndromes: a cross-sectional lstudy. BMC Geriatr 2022;22:157.
28. Palatini P, Mos L, Rattazzi M, et al. Blood pressure response to standing is a strong determinant of masked hypertension in young to middle-age individuals. J Hypertens 2022;40:1927–34.
29. Kario K. Orthostatic hypertension-a new haemodynamic cardiovascular risk factor. Nat Rev Nephrol 2013;9:726–38.
30. Robertson D, Hollister AS, Biaggioni I, et al. The diagnosis and treatment of baroreflex failure. N Engl J Med 1993;329:1449–55.
31. Heusser K, Tank J, Luft FC, et al. Baroreflex failure. Hypertension 2005;45:834–9.
32. Biaggioni I, Shibao CA, Diedrich A, et al. Blood pressure management in afferent baroreflex failure: JACC review topic of the week. J Am Coll Cardiol 2019;74:2939–47.
33. Norcliffe-Kaufmann L, Axelrod F, Kaufmann H. Afferent baroreflex failure in familial dysautonomia. Neurology 2010;75:1904–11.
34. Fanciulli A, Jordan J, Biaggioni I, et al. Consensus statement on the definition of neurogenic supine hypertension in cardiovascular autonomic failure by the American autonomic Society (AAS) and the European Federation of autonomic Societies (EFAS): Endorsed by the European Academy of Neurology (EAN) and the European Society of hypertension (ESH). Clin Auton Res 2018;28:355–62.
35. Golden EP, Vernino S. Autoimmune autonomic neuropathies and ganglionopathies: epidemiology, pathophysiology, and therapeutic advances. Clin Auton Res 2019;29:277–88.
36. Wieling W, Kaufmann H, Claydon VE, et al. Diagnosis and treatment of orthostatic hypotension. Lancet Neurol 2022;21:735–46.
37. Jordan J, Fanciulli A, Tank J, et al. Management of supine hypertension in patients with neurogenic orthostatic hypotension: scientific statement of the American Autonomic Society, European Federation of Autonomic Societies, and the European Society of Hypertension. J Hypertens 2019;37:1541–6.

38. Mancia G, Facchetti R, Bombelli M, et al. White-coat hypertension: pathophysiological and clinical aspects: Excellence award for hypertension Research 2020. Hypertension 2021;78:1677–88.

39. Cohen JB, Lotito MJ, Trivedi UK, et al. Cardiovascular events and mortality in white coat hypertension: a systematic review and meta-analysis. Ann Intern Med 2019;170:853–62.

40. Stergiou GS, Asayama K, Thijs L, et al. International Database on HOme blood pressure in relation to Cardiovascular Outcome (IDHOCO) Investigators. Prognosis of white-coat and masked hypertension: International Database of HOme blood pressure in relation to Cardiovascular Outcome. Hypertension 2014;63:675–82.

41. Anstey DE, Muntner P, Bello NA, et al. Diagnosing masked hypertension using ambulatory blood pressure monitoring, home blood pressure monitoring, or both? Hypertension 2018;72:1200.

42. Thakkar HV, Pope A, Anpalahan M. Masked hypertension: a systematic review. Heart Lung Circ 2020;29:102–11.

43. Korzets A, Korzets Z, Zingerman B. Pseudohypertension in the very elderly: important or not? Isr Med Assoc J 2023;25:68–9.

44. AlGhatrif M, Wang M, Fedorova OV, et al. The pressure of aging. Med Clin North Am 2017;101:81–101.

45. Weinstein JR, Anderson S. The aging kidney: physiological changes. Adv Chronic Kidney Dis 2010;17:302–7.

46. Cowley AW Jr, Mattson DL, LU S, et al. The renal medulla in hypertension. Hypertension 1995;25:663–73.

47. Mau T, Yung R. Adipose tissue inflammation in aging. Exp Gerontol 2018;105:27–31.

48. Hunter GR, Gower BA, Kane BL. Age related shift in visceral fat. Int J Body Compos Res 2010;8:103–8.

49. Vogt L, Marques FZ, Fujita T, et al. Novel mechanisms of salt-sensitive hypertension. Kid Internat 2023;104:690–7.

50. Whelton PK, Appel LJ, Espeland MA, et al. Sodium reduction and weight loss in the treatment of hypertension in older persons: a randomized control trials of nonpharmacologic interventions in the elderly (TONE). JAMA 1998;279:839–46.

51. Rockwood K, Song X, MacKnight C, et al. A global clinical measure of fitness and frailty in elderly people. CMAJ (Can Med Assoc J) 2005;173:489–95.

52. Katz S. Assessing self-maintenance: activities of daily living, mobility and instrumental activities of daily living. JAGS 1983;31:721–6.

53. Zygouris S, Tsolaki M. Computerized cognitive testing for older adults: a review. Am J Alzheimer's Dis Other Dementias 2015;30:13–28.

54. Schwandt A, Denkinger M, Fasching P, et al. Comparison of MDRD, CKD-EPI, and Cockcroft-Gault equation in relation to measured glomerular filtration rate among a large cohort with diabetes. J Diab Complic 2017;31:1376–83.

55. Willems JM, Vlasveld T, den Elzen WPJ, et al. Performance of Cockcroft-Gault, MDRD, and CKD-EPI in estimating prevalence of renal function and predicting survival in the oldest old. BMC Geriatr 2013;13:113.

56. Gottlieb DJ, Punjabi NM. Diagnosis and management of obstructive sleep apnea: a review. JAMA 2020;323:1389–400.

57. Badr MS, Dingell JD, Javaheri S. Central sleep apnea: a brief review. Curr Pulmonol Rep 2019;8:14–21.

58. Chung F, Yegneswaran B, Liao P, et al. STOP Questionnaire: a tool to screen patients for obstructive sleep apnea. Anesthesiology 2008;108:812–21.

59. Carey RM, Calhoun D, Bakris G, et al. Resistant hypertension: detection, evaluation and management. A scientific statement from the American Heart Association. Hypertension 2018;72:e53–90.
60. Sarathy H, Salman LA, Lee C, et al. Evaluation and management of secondary hypertension. Med Clin North Am 2022;106:269–83.
61. Chrysochou C, Foley RN, Young JF, et al. Dispelling the myth: the use of renin-angiotensin blockade in atheromatous renovascular disease. Nephrol Dial Transplant 2012;27:1403.
62. Conn JW, Louis LH. Primary aldosteronism: a new clinical entity. Trans Assoc Am Physicians 1955;68:215–31 [discussion: 231–3].
63. Hughes D, Judge C, Murphy R, et al. Association of blood pressure lowering with incident dementia or cognitive impairment: a systematic review and meta-analysis. JAMA 2020;323:1934–44.
64. Supiano MA. Optimal blood pressure targets with age. Clin Geriatr Med 2024;40(4).
65. Five-year findings of the hypertension detection and follow-up program. II. Mortality by race-sex and age. Hypertension Detection and Follow-up Program Cooperative Group. JAMA 1979;7(242):2572–7.
66. The Australian National Blood Pressure Study. A therapeutic trial in mild hypertension. Aust Fam Physician 1981;10(234):237–9.
67. Amery A, Birkenhäger W, Brixko P, et al. Mortality and morbidity results from the European working party on high blood pressure in the elderly trial. Lancet 1985; 1(8442):1349–54.
68. Coope J, Warrender TS. Randomised trial of treatment of hypertension in elderly patients in primary care. Br Med J 1986;293:1145–51.
69. Dahlöf B, Lindholm LH, Hansson L, et al. Morbidity and mortality in the Swedish trial in old patients with hypertension (STOP-Hypertension). Lancet 1991;338: 1281–5.
70. Prevention of stroke by antihypertensive drug treatment in older persons with isolated systolic hypertension. Final results of the systolic hypertension in the elderly program (SHEP). SHEP Cooperative Research group. JAMA 1991;265: 3255–64.
71. Medical Research Council trial of treatment of hypertension in older adults: principal results. MRC Working Party. BMJ 1992;304:405–12.
72. Gong L, Zhang W, Zhu Y, et al. Shanghai trial of nifedipine in the elderly (STONE). J Hypertens 1996;14:1237–45.
73. Staessen JA, Fagard R, Thijs L, et al. Randomised double-blind comparison of placebo and active treatment for older patients with isolated systolic hypertension. The Systolic Hypertension in Europe (Syst-Eur) Trial Investigators. Lancet 1997;350:757–64.
74. Wang J-G, Staeseen JA, Gong L, et al. For the Systolic Hypertension in China (Syst-China) Collaborative Group: Chinese trial on isolated systolic hypertension in the elderly. Arch Intern Med 2000;160:211–20.
75. Wing LM, Reid CM, Ryan P, et al, Second Australian National Blood Pressure Study Group. A comparison of outcomes with angiotensin-converting–enzyme inhibitors and diuretics for hypertension in the elderly. NEJM 2003;348:583–92.
76. Beckett NS, Peters R, Fletcher AE, et al, HYVET Study Group. Treatment of hypertension in patients 80 years of age or older. NEJM 2008;358:1887–98.
77. Williamson JD, Supiano MA, Applegate WB, et al, SPRINT Research Group. Intensive vs standard blood pressure control and cardiovascular disease

outcomes in adults aged ≥75 years: a Randomized Clinical Trial. JAMA 2016; 315(24):2673–82.

78. Kitagawa K, Yamamoto Y, Arima H, et al, Recurrent Stroke Prevention Clinical Outcome (RESPECT) Study Group. Effect of standard vs intensive blood pressure control on the risk of recurrent stroke: a randomized clinical trial and meta-analysis. JAMA Neurol 2019;76:1309–18.

79. Zhang W, Zhang S, Deng Y, et al, for the STEP Study Group. Trial of intensive blood-pressure control in older patients with hypertension. NEJM 2021;385: 1268–79.

80. de Havenon A, et al. Cognitive function and blood pressure in older adults. Clin Geriatr Med 2024;40(4).

81. Weinberger MH, Fineberg NS. Sodium and volume sensitivity of blood pressure: age and pressure change over time. Hypertension 1991;18:67–71.

82. Moore TJ, Conlin PR, Ard J, et al. DASH (Dietary Approaches to Stop Hypertension) Diet is effective treatment for stage 1 isolated systolic hypertension. Hypertension 2001;38:155–8.

83. Filippou CD, Tsioufis CP, Thomopoulos CG, et al. Dietary Approaches to Stop Hypertension (DASH) Diet and blood pressure reduction in adults with and without hypertension: a systematic review and meta-analysis of randomized controlled trials. Adv Nutr 2020;11:1150–60.

84. Jennings A, Berendsen AM, de Groot LCPGM, et al. Mediterranean-style diet improves systolic blood pressure and arterial stiffness in olde adults: results of a 1-year European multi-center trial. Hypertension 2019;73:578–86.

85. Trichopoulou A, Vasilopoulou E. Mediterranean diet and longevity. Brit J Nutr 2000;84(S2):S205–9.

86. Colleluori G, Villareal DT. Aging, obesity, sarcopenia and the effect of diet and exercise intervention. Exp Gerontol 2021;155:111561.

87. Kazeminia M, Daneshkhah A, Jalali R, et al. The effect of exercise on older adult's blood pressure suffering hypertension: systematic review and meta-analysis on clinical trial studies. Int J Hypertension 2020. https://doi.org/10.1155/2020/2786120.

88. Dempsey PC, Sacre JW, Larsen RN, et al. Interrupting prolonged sitting with brief bouts of light walking or simple resistance activities reduces resting blood pressure and plasma noradrenaline in type 2 diabetes. J Hypertension 2016;34: 2376–82.

89. Egan BM. Are there cardiometabolic benefits of low-intensity physical activity in at-risk adults? JASH 2018;12:69–70.

90. Thomopoulos C. Target blood pressure in isolated systolic hypertension. A meta-analysis of randomized outcome trials. J Hypertension 2023;41:2113–4.

91. Thomopoulos C, Parati G, Zanchetti A. Effects of blood pressure-lowering treatment on cardiovascular outcomes and mortality: 13 - benefits and adverse events in older and younger patients with hypertension: overview, meta-analyses and meta-regression analyses of randomized trials. J Hypertension 2018;36:1622–36.

92. Brunstrom M, Carlberg B, Kjeldsen SE. Effect of antihypertensive treatment in isolated systolic hypertension (ISH) - systematic review and meta-analysis of randomised controlled trials. Blood Press 2023;32:2226757.

93. Egan BM, Kjeldsen SE, Narkiewicz K, et al. Single-pill combinations, hypertension control and clinical outcomes: potential, pitfalls and solutions. Blood Pres 2022;31:164–8.

94. Benetos A, Rossignol P, Cherubini A, et al. Polypharmacy in the aging patient: management of hypertension in octogenarians. JAMA 2015;314:170–80.

95. Pajewski NM, Berlowitz DR, Bress AP, et al. Intensive vs standard blood pressure control in adults 80 Years or older: a secondary analysis of the systolic blood pressure intervention trial. J Am Geriatr Soc 2020;68:496–504.
96. Warwick J, Falaschetti E, Rockwood K, et al. No evidence that frailty modifies the positive impact of antihypertensive treatment in very elderly people: an investigation of the impact of frailty upon treatment effect in the HYpertension in the Very Elderly Trial (HYVET) study, a double-blind, placebo-controlled study of antihypertensives in people with hypertension aged 80 and over. BMC Med 2015;13:78.
97. Odden MC, Peralta CA, Haan MN, et al. Rethinking the association of high blood pressure with mortality in elderly adults: the impact of frailty. Arch Intern Med 2012;72:1162–8.
98. Kremer KM, Braisch U, Rothenbacher D, et al. Systolic blood pressure and mortality in community-dwelling older adults: frailty as an effect modifier. Hypertension 2022;79:24–32.
99. Riemer TG, Villagomez Fuentes LE, Algharably EAE, et al. Do β-blockers cause depression? Systematic review and meta-analysis of psychiatric adverse events during β-blocker therapy. Hypertension 2021;77:1539–48.
100. Wilcox CS. Antihypertensive and renal mechanisms of SGLT2 (sodium-glucose linked transport 2) inhibitors. Hypertension 2020;75:894–901.
101. Ferdinand KC, Izzo JL, Lee J, et al. Antihyperglycmie and blood pressure effects of empagliflozin in black patients with type 2 diabetes mellitus and hypertension. Circulation 2019;139:2098–109.
102. Kario K, Ferdinand KC, Vongpatanasin W. Are SGLT2 inhibitors new hypertension drugs? Circulation 2021;143:1750–3.
103. Huggett RJ, Scott EM, Gilbey SG, et al. Impact of type 2 diabetes mellitus on sympathetic neural mechanisms in hypertension. Circulation 2003;108:3097–101.
104. Beal B, Schutte AE, Neuen BL. Blood pressure effects of SGLT2 inhibitors: mechanisms and clinical evidence in different populations. Curr Hypertension Rep 2023;25:429–35.
105. Ambaradekar AV, Sailer C. SGLT2 inhibitors and blood pressure in heart failure. JACC (J Am Coll Cardiol) 2023;11:90–2.
106. Vongpatanasin W, Giacona JM. Resistant hypertension in older adults. Clin Geriatr Med 2024;40(4).
107. Swaminathan R, East C, Feldman D, et al. SCAI Position Statement on Renal Denervation for Hypertension: patient selection, operator competence, training and techniques, and organizational recommendations. J Soc Cardiov Angiog Interv 2023;2:101121.
108. Fengler K, Rommel KP, Lapusca R, et al. Renal denervation in isolated systolic hypertension using different catheter techniques and technologies. Hypertension 2019;74(2):341–8.
109. Salah HM, Fudim M. Barostim baroreflex activation therapy: expert analysis. ACC. 02 Dec 2022. Available at: https://www.acc.org/Latest-in-Cardiology/Articles/2022/2/02/13/14/Barostim-Baroflex-Activation-Therapy (accessed 22 Feb 2024).
110. Petriceks AH, Appel LJ, Miller ER 3rd, et al. Timing of orthostatic hypotension and its relationship with falls in older adults. J Am Geriatr Soc 2023;71:3711–20.
111. Benetos A, Bulpitt CJ, Petrovic M, et al. An expert opinion from the European Society of hypertension/European union Geriatric medicine Society working group on the management of hypertension in very old, frail Subjects. Hypertension 2016;67:820–5.
112. Applegate WB, Williamson JD, Berlowitz D. Deprescribing antihypertensive medication in elderly adults. JAMA 2020;324:1682.

Long-term Monitoring of Blood Pressure in Older Adults

A Focus on Self-Measured Blood Pressure Monitoring

Collin Burks, MD[a],*, Daichi Shimbo, MD[b],
Christopher Barrett Bowling, MD, MSPH[c]

KEYWORDS

- Hypertension • Self-measured blood pressure • Older adults

KEY POINTS

- Self-measured blood pressure (SMBP) monitoring is a practical method for out-of-office blood pressure measurement.
- SMBP monitoring is an evidence-based strategy to improve BP control in hypertension management.
- Older adults may face unique challenges in conducting SMBP monitoring yet stand to benefit the most.

INTRODUCTION

Hypertension is among the most common chronic conditions in older adults with a prevalence of over 70% among US adults aged 65 years or older.[1] Among older adults, hypertension treatment is known to be effective, reducing the risk of cardiovascular disease events.[2] However, despite these known benefits, most older US adults with hypertension do not achieve the guideline-recommended blood pressure (BP) control.[3] Recent reports have shown that the percentage of older adults with BP control has declined over the last decade,[4] resulting in calls for renewed efforts to improve BP control in this population.[5,6]

[a] Department of Medicine, Duke University School of Medicine, 4220 North Roxboro Street, Durham, NC 27704 USA; [b] Department of Medicine, Columbia University Irving Medical Center, 60 Haven Avenue, Office Suite B234, New York, NY 10032, USA; [c] Durham Veterans Affairs Geriatric Research Education and Clinical Center, Durham Veterans Affairs Medical Center (VAMC), 508 Fulton Street, Durham, NC 27705, USA
* Corresponding author.
E-mail address: collin.burks@duke.edu

Clin Geriatr Med 40 (2024) 573–583
https://doi.org/10.1016/j.cger.2024.04.009
0749-0690/24/© 2024 Elsevier Inc. All rights reserved.

One recommended strategy for improving BP control among older adults is to increase the use of out-of-office BP monitoring.[6–8] The advantages and challenges of out-of-office BP monitoring among older adults have not been extensively reported. In this review, we discuss approaches to long-term monitoring of BP among older adults, with a focus on self-measured BP (SMBP) monitoring at home. We first describe home BP monitoring (HBPM) options and discuss their indications. We then present evidence for HBPM, focusing on the SMBP monitoring approach and ways to optimize its use. Next, we consider the unique benefits of SMBP monitoring for older adults before moving on to a discussion of the specific challenges older adults may face with SMBP monitoring. We conclude by discussing how to address the challenges at multiple levels and by providing recommendations for clinical care of older adults with hypertension.

OUT-OF-OFFICE BLOOD PRESSURE MONITORING
Definitions

BP monitoring can occur in health care settings, community settings, and the home. Out-of-office BP measurement refers to all measurements taken outside of a health care setting, including ambulatory BP monitoring (ABPM) and SMBP monitoring. ABPM is a specific method of obtaining BP measurements over a set amount of time, typically 24 hours.[9] In ABPM, an individual wears a fully automated BP monitor, along with a cuff on the upper arm, and participates in their daily life as BP measurements are taken on a set interval period. SMBP monitoring refers to individuals taking their own BP at home with a semiautomated, oscillometric device. While this term is often used interchangeably with the term "home BP monitoring," "self-measured" emphasizes the role of the patient in this method. Therefore, we will use the term SMBP monitoring to describe this method of self-monitoring of BP at home.

Indications and Evidence

Guidelines from the American College of Cardiology/American Heart Association recommend the use of out-of-office BP measurements to confirm a diagnosis of hypertension, as well as to guide medication titration for lowering of BP.[1] Other indications for out-of-office BP measurement include screening for white coat hypertension, in which BP is elevated in office but normal outside of office, and masked hypertension, in which BP is normal in office but elevated outside of office.[1,9] Out-of-office BP measurement is also indicated in detecting white coat effect, in which people on medications for hypertension have elevated BP in office but controlled BP outside of the office, and masked uncontrolled hypertension, in which people on medications for hypertension have controlled BP in office but elevated BP outside of the office.[1,9] Additionally, ABPM or SMBP monitoring can be utilized for detection of the transition from white coat hypertension to sustained hypertension, while ABPM may be useful for confirming high readings in scenarios such as masked uncontrolled hypertension or white coat effect.[1] Several international guidelines for hypertension include recommendations that SMBP monitoring is used to improve medication adherence.[7]

Compared to in-office BP measurements, SMBP has been found to better predict outcomes, such as cardiovascular mortality and call-cause mortality.[10] It also better predicts end-organ damage, such as proteinuria, compared to office BP.[6] Additionally, SMBP monitoring has been shown to improve adherence to medications.[11] However, SMBP monitoring alone, without any other co-intervention such as standardized medication titration or lifestyle counseling, has modest impact on lowering BP.[12] A meta-analysis by Tucker and colleagues found that SMBP monitoring interventions which include 1:1 support for patients and medication intensification were more successful at lowering BP in comparison to SMBP monitoring alone.[12] Finally, compared to ABPM, SMBP monitoring is typically easier to implement and more widely available.[1]

Protocols for Conducting Self-measured Blood Pressure

Protocols and procedures for SMBP monitoring have been developed to guide patients and clinicians to successfully conduct SMBP.[1] For SMBP monitoring to improve hypertension management, BP measures need to be accurate, conducted at an appropriate interval, and communicated to providers. For example, in a study focused on increasing SMBP monitoring across the United States, Wall and colleagues describe optimal SMBP monitoring as including a feedback loop in which patients and clinicians work together via remote data exchange.[13] Ideally, with assistance from the health care team, patients with hypertension are first trained to (1) choose a validated monitoring device and correct cuff size, (2) properly prepare and position themselves for a reading, (3) follow a monitoring protocol, and (4) transmit data back to their clinical team. After a patient uses SMBP monitoring, their clinical team interprets the data received and sends recommendations to the patient, and the cycle continues.

Standard protocols for monitoring frequency recommend that individuals take 2 measurements in both morning and evening, for at least 3 days and a preferred period up to 7 days.[7] As less frequent measurement could improve adherence with SMBP monitoring, studies have attempted to identify the ideal frequency for monitoring. One study found that 3 days of monitoring may be enough to identify or exclude elevated BP in most patients.[14] For people with stable, controlled BPs, the frequency of monitoring can decrease to 1 to 3 days every week or month.[7,8]

Use of Self-measured Blood Pressure by Older Adults

Estimates of how often SMBP monitoring is used among older adults have been shown to vary. Although a large percentage of older adults report measuring their BP at home, reporting the results to their health care providers is much less common. For example, one study that surveyed nearly 67,000 adults aged 65 years and older who had hypertension found that 65% of respondents reported checking their BP outside the office (90% at home).[15] However, only 4% of those people reported sharing their measurements with a health care professional via email or over the Internet. This absence of transmission may reduce the likelihood that SMBP monitoring leads to changes in hypertension treatment or improve BP control. In a separate study of 1050 US adults aged 50 to 80 years with diagnosed hypertension, 51% reported regularly monitoring their BP.[16] In this study, 77% of those with hypertension reported having a home BP monitor device with an arm cuff, and 51% shared their readings with a health professional. Of those with hypertension who did not have a home device, reasons given by the respondents included they never thought about getting one or devices were too expensive (**Fig. 1**). These findings suggest areas for improvement in helping patients obtain a device, report results to providers, and understand the importance of monitoring.

BENEFITS OF SELF-MEASURED BLOOD PRESSURE FOR OLDER ADULTS

There are several reasons to believe that older adults might benefit the most from widespread use of SMBP monitoring. With the highest rates of hypertension and multiple chronic conditions, many older adults may stand to benefit significantly from achieving lower BP goals and sustaining BP control that occurs with SMBP

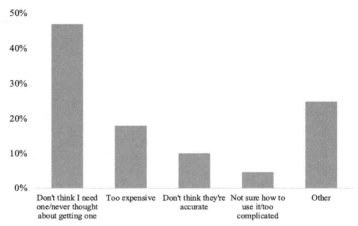

Fig. 1. Percentage of respondents with hypertension, without a home device, who gave the abovementioned reasons for not having a home blood pressure monitor device. (*Data from* Springer MV, Malani P, Solway E, et al. Prevalence and Frequency of Self-measured Blood Pressure Monitoring in US Adults Aged 50–80 Years. JAMA Netw Open. Sep 1 2022;5(9):e2231772. https://doi.org/10.1001/jamanetworkopen.2022.31772)

monitoring. Sustained BP control has been shown to be associated with a lower the risk for outcomes that are important to older adults, including progression of multimorbidity and nursing home admission.[17–19] Additionally, older adults with mobility challenges, transportation challenges, or other barriers to traditional in-office care could benefit from the need for fewer office visits with use of SMBP monitoring.[20] Although not well studied to date, it is also likely that SMBP monitoring could be used to avoid hypotension related to overtreatment of hypertension and lower the risk of falls. Prior studies have shown the risk of serious fall injuries to be highest in the 2 weeks following the initiation or intensification of a hypertension medication.[21] The use of SMBP monitoring may also help indirectly decrease social isolation, common in older adults,[22] by facilitating more contact with their health care providers, and it may increase self-efficacy in older adults.[23] While more research is needed to evaluate possible benefits, SMBP monitoring may contribute to improving equity in hypertension care.[24]

CHALLENGES IN SELF-MEASURED BLOOD PRESSURE FOR OLDER POPULATIONS
General Implementation Challenges

Challenges to successful implementation of SMBP monitoring for the general population are numerous and can be described as patient-, clinician-, and health care system-level barriers. At the patient level, difficulties can include obtaining a validated BP cuff, utilizing the proper cuff size, and following the correct technique and monitoring schedule.[25] At the clinician level, health care professionals may lack the training and time to teach patients how to initiate HBPM and to respond to the patient-generated data.[26] In addition, clinicians may not be aware of the 2 current procedural terminology (CPT) codes that exist to provide reimbursement for clinician services related to out-of-office BP monitoring.[13] At the systems level, there may be a lack of support for team-based clinical care, which has been shown to be effective in managing hypertension.[27] Without standardized protocols and workflows, SMBP monitoring can be hard for health care systems to scale. In addition, electronic health records (EHRs) may not have the capability to efficiently display the data for clinicians.[28]

In addition to the challenges discussed earlier, there are unique challenges that older adults may face (**Fig. 2**). We will describe some of these potential challenges later. However, older adults are not a monolithic group, and it is important to note that not all of these challenges necessarily apply to each older adult.

Challenges Translating Published Research Findings to Older Adults

A major challenge to applying evidence-based clinical practice guideline recommendations, such as those encouraging SMBP monitoring, to geriatric populations is the underrepresentation of older adults in the clinical trials used in evidence synthesis.[29] Underrepresentation of older adults in research occurs when clinical trials set upper age cutoffs, apply exclusions that disproportionately affect older adults such as co-morbidity, or when research teams fail to address known barriers to research participation. Underrepresentation relative to the population prevalence of hypertension is common in cardiovascular disease research. For example, a report addressing the rationale for the National Institutes of Health (NIH) inclusion across the life span policy showed that adults aged 75 years or older accounted for less than 5% of all adults enrolled into NIH-funded hypertension research studies in 2021.[30] This is despite that individuals 75 years and older comprise nearly 20% of the US adult population with hypertension. More specific to SMBP studies, the meta-analysis on SMBP monitoring by Tucker and colleagues found that 21% of participants were aged 70 to

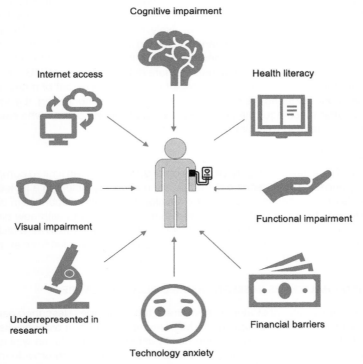

Fig. 2. Selected potential challenges in self-measured blood pressure monitoring for older adults.

79 years and only 7% were aged 80 years or above.[12] Further limiting our ability to assess the generalizability of research on SMBP monitoring is the lack of information on the prevalence of physical function, sensory limitations, and cognitive impairment in the study populations, all of which may impact an older adult's ability to use SMBP monitoring, as we discuss later.

Health-related Challenges

Older adults are more likely to experience health conditions such as arthritis, lymphedema, and visual impairment that could make manipulating and wearing BP monitoring devices more difficult. The presence of cognitive impairment, the risk of which increases with advancing age, may also make it more difficult for individuals to successfully use monitoring devices and engage in SMBP monitoring. Older adults with functional or cognitive impairments might have to rely on help from a care partner, who may not be available, have the training, or be willing to assist with SMBP monitoring.

The development of new health conditions and declining life expectancy for older adults may alter the decision to use SMBP monitoring. For example, the discovery of a terminal cancer or progression of dementia may shift an individual's health priorities and negate the need for strictly controlled BP or their desire to engage in SMBP monitoring.

Challenges due to Social Determinants of Health

Social determinants of health (SDOH) that negatively impact patients can also pose challenges to successful use of SMBP monitoring. For example, financial barriers, which are common in older adults,[31] may prohibit the purchase of BP monitoring devices. Additionally, older adults are more likely to have lower health literacy than younger or middle-aged adults,[32] potentially making it more difficult for them to understand and follow a BP monitoring schedule. Twenty-five percent of older adults do not have Internet access,[13] which could make remote data exchange in SMBP monitoring difficult or impossible. These examples depict just a few ways, out of many, in which SDOH may impact older adults capacity to conduct SMBP monitoring. It is important to recognize that these age-related SDOH are magnified in persons who experience health inequities related to structural racism.[24]

Technology-related Challenges

The adoption of digital health technology by older adults has been limited compared to other age groups.[33] The reasons behind this are numerous, including a lack of attention to needs of older adults in technology development[33] and disparities in digital literacy. Older adults are more likely to report that they need help with new electronic devices,[34] and some have technology anxiety as well as concerns over a lack of privacy.[20] These technology-related concerns may deter an older adult from engaging in a process of remote data exchange.

ADDRESSING CHALLENGES IN SELF-MEASURED BLOOD PRESSURE

There are several potential strategies to address the challenges described earlier and facilitate more widespread adoption of SMBP monitoring among older adults. These strategies can occur at the clinician and health care system levels, as well as at the societal level. For example, clinicians and health care systems can provide more education to patients and caregivers about the importance of SMBP monitoring for those with hypertension. In addition, clinicians can be taught how to train patients and their caregivers to properly conduct SMBP monitoring.[35] Health care systems can use re-sources, such as those from the Million Hearts initiative,[36] to incorporate new proto-cols and workflows for SMBP monitoring implementation. Health care systems can also partner with local institutions, such as senior centers and local Y associations, to increase education around SMBP monitoring.[13,28] At the societal level, increasing access to high-speed Internet may help overcome some barriers to use of SMBP monitoring.[13] In addition to increasing Internet access, increasing access to techno-logical support may be beneficial.[13] Finally, the development of new BP monitoring devices that do not rely on manual dexterity could benefit older adults, as could increasing inclusion of older adults in research studies. These strategies, and more, are possible long-term strategies to increase the use of SMBP monitoring in older adults.

There are also several short-term strategies to increase the adoption and usefulness of SMBP monitoring in older populations. For example, an assessment of an older adult's strengths and challenges as they relate to using SMBP monitoring may help the clinician, patient, and caregiver work together to develop a practical, individualized BP monitoring plan. This process could be guided by the geriatrics 5Ms (Mind, Med-ications, Mobility, Multicomplexity, and Matters Most) in the clinical setting (**Table 1**). This framework may aid the clinician in identifying the conditions that could impact an older adult's ability to successfully utilize and benefit from SMBP monitoring. In this framework, we also suggest solutions to overcome potential barriers.

Mind

The clinician should be aware of whether the patient has any cognitive impairment that may impact their ability to understand and follow an SMBP monitoring plan. Addition-ally, inquiring about previous use of technology and digital literacy may be helpful as is knowing whether there are any concerns about health literacy. If barriers are encoun-tered, solutions may include involving a family member or referring to a local senior center for a class on chronic disease management.

Medications

The clinician should inquire about medication adherence and assess the complexity of a patient's medication regimen. If medication issues are encountered, education from the clinician might help, as could simplifying a regimen or referring to a pharmacist. Encouraging use of a pillbox or blister pack from a pharmacy may be important in some circumstances.

Mobility

Understanding whether a patient is functionally independent or requires assistance with certain activities of daily life may give information as to what help, if any, an older adult might need in using SMBP monitoring. Involving family might be helpful, as could referring to physical therapy or occupational therapy to work on any functional challenges.

Multicomplexity

Considering the complexity of the health and social situations of individual patients is important. As it relates to SMBP monitoring, knowing whether the patient has visual impairment that could impact their ability to use a BP monitor is important. In addition, understanding the other chronic conditions the patient has may help the clinician give specific guidance on initiating SMBP monitoring. Finally, assessing SDOH, such as financial barriers, may lead to a more feasible treatment plan. Potential solutions within

Table 1
Applying the geriatric 5Ms framework to improve the use of self-measured blood pressure monitoring among older adults

Geriatric 5Ms	Challenges to SBMP	Strategies to Improve SMBP Monitoring
Mind	• Cognitive impairment • Low health literacy • Low digital literacy	• Involve family/care partner(s) • Referral to educator • Referral to community resources for classes • Simplify monitoring schedule
Medications	• Complex medication regimen • Low medication adherence • Cost	• Education • Simplify regimen • Referral to pharmacist • Encourage use of pillbox or pack
Mobility	• Functional limitations (ADLs, IADLs) • Dexterity • Fall risk	• Involve family/care partner(s) • Referral to PT and/or OT
Multicomplexity	• Visual impairment • Multiple chronic conditions • Financial challenges	• Involve family/care partner(s) • Consider alternatives to upper arm cuff • Referral to PT and/or OT • Referral to social worker • Provide BP loaner device
Matters Most	• Goals and priorities • Limited life expectancy	• Align intervention with goals • Motivational interviewing • Involve family/care partner(s)

Abbreviations: ADLs, activities of daily living; IADLs, instrumental activities of daily living; OT, occupational therapy; PT, physical therapy.

this realm include involving a family member, providing a BP monitor (if a loaner program is available) or referring to a social worker for connection to resources.

Matters Most

The clinician should assess each patient's goals and priorities as it relates to management of their BP. If controlling BP is already a significant priority for the patient, designing an SMBP monitoring plan may not take much effort. If the patient does not see BP control as a priority, the clinician may need to delve further into the patient's goals and discuss how SMBP may align with their goals. Motivational interviewing may be helpful, as could family member involvement. Finally, considering the person's life expectancy may help direct goals and treatment plans for hypertension.

SUMMARY

Long-term monitoring of BP is a key component of hypertension treatment and control. SMBP monitoring, a practical out-of-office method for long-term monitoring of BP, has been shown to be beneficial for BP control. Older adults, who have the highest prevalence of hypertension, might face the most significant challenges in using SMBP monitoring but may reap the greatest benefits. Barriers to widespread implementation of SMBP monitoring must be addressed from the individual to societal level. Clinically, understanding an older adult's unique challenges and opportunities will help the clinician tailor an individualized plan for SMBP monitoring.

CLINICS CARE POINTS

- A toolkit for SMBP monitoring implementation is available on the Million Heart Initiative's Web site, along with numerous other resources for patients, clinicians, and health care systems.[36]
- Older adults should be counseled on the recommended frequency and duration of BP measurements at home.
- Older adults should use a validated BP device to measure their BP at home. A list of validated devices is available at: https://www.validatebp.org [37]
- Understanding the unique challenges and opportunities of the older adult in front of you will help you tailor an SMBP monitoring intervention beneficial to them.

DISCLOSURE

The authors have nothing to disclose.

REFERENCES

1. Whelton PK, Carey RM, Aronow WS, et al. 2017 ACC/AHA/AAPA/ABC/ACPM/AGS/APhA/ASH/ASPC/NMA/PCNA guideline for the prevention, detection, evaluation, and management of high blood pressure in adults: executive summary: a report of the american college of cardiology/american heart association task force on clinical practice guidelines. Circulation 2018;138(17):e426–83.
2. Pharmacological blood pressure lowering for primary and secondary prevention of cardiovascular disease across different levels of blood pressure: an individual participant-level data meta-analysis. Lancet 2021;397(10285):1625–36.
3. Centers for Disease Control and Prevention. Hypertension cascade: hypertension prevalence, treatment and control estimates among us adults aged 18 years and older applying the criteria from the american college of cardiology and american heart association's 2017 hypertension guideline—NHANES 2017–2020. 2023. Available at: https://millionhearts.hhs.gov/data-reports/hypertension-prevalence.html. [Accessed 29 January 2024].
4. Muntner P, Miles MA, Jaeger BC, et al. Blood pressure control among us adults, 2009 to 2012 through 2017 to 2020. Hypertension 2022;79(9):1971–80.
5. U.S. Department of Health and Human Services. The surgeon general's call to action to control hypertension. 2020. Available at: https://www.cdc.gov/bloodpressure/docs/SG-CTA-HTN-Control-Report-508.pdf. [Accessed 29 January 2024].
6. Abdalla M, Bolen SD, Brettler J, et al. Implementation strategies to improve blood pressure control in the United States: a scientific statement from the american heart association and american medical association. Hypertension 2023;80(10):e143–57.
7. Shimbo D, Artinian NT, Basile JN, et al. Self-measured blood pressure monitoring at home: a joint policy statement from the american heart association and american medical association. Circulation 2020;142(4):e42–63.

8. Unger T, Borghi C, Charchar F, et al. 2020 International society of hypertension global hypertension practice guidelines. Hypertension 2020;75(6):1334–57.

9. Reynolds K, Bowling CB, Sim JJ, et al. The utility of ambulatory blood pressure monitoring for diagnosing white coat hypertension in older adults. Curr Hypertens Rep 2015;17(11):86.

10. Fuchs SC, Mello RG, Fuchs FC. Home blood pressure monitoring is better predictor of cardiovascular disease and target organ damage than office blood pressure: a systematic review and meta-analysis. Curr Cardiol Rep 2013;15(11):413.

11. Fletcher BR, Hartmann-Boyce J, Hinton L, et al. The effect of self-monitoring of blood pressure on medication adherence and lifestyle factors: a systematic review and meta-analysis. Am J Hypertens 2015;28(10):1209–21.

12. Tucker KL, Sheppard JP, Stevens R, et al. Self-monitoring of blood pressure in hypertension: a systematic review and individual patient data meta-analysis. PLoS Med 2017;14(9):e1002389.

13. Wall HK, Wright JS, Jackson SL, et al. How do we jump-start self-measured blood pressure monitoring in the United States? addressing barriers beyond the published literature. Am J Hypertens 2022;35(3):244–55.

14. Bradley CK, Choi E, Abdalla M, et al. Use of different blood pressure thresholds to reduce the number of home blood pressure monitoring days needed for detecting hypertension. Hypertension 2023;80(10):2169–77.

15. Fang J, Luncheon C, Wall HK, et al. Self-measured blood pressure monitoring among adults with self-reported hypertension in 20 us states and the District of Columbia, 2019. Am J Hypertens 2021;34(11):1148–53.

16. Springer MV, Malani P, Solway E, et al. Prevalence and frequency of self-measured blood pressure monitoring in US adults aged 50-80 years. JAMA Netw Open 2022;5(9):e2231772.

17. Bowling CB, Sloane R, Pieper C, et al. Sustained SBP control and long-term nursing home admission among Medicare beneficiaries. J Hypertens 2021;39(11):2258–64.

18. Bowling CB, Lee A, Williamson JD. Blood pressure control among older adults with hypertension: narrative review and introduction of a framework for improving care. Am J Hypertens 2021;34(3):258–66.

19. Bowling CB, Sloane R, Pieper C, et al. Association of sustained blood pressure control with multimorbidity progression among older adults. J Am Geriatr Soc 2020;68(9):2059–66.

20. Searcy RP, Summapund J, Estrin D, et al. Mobile health technologies for older adults with cardiovascular disease: current evidence and future directions. Current Geriatrics Reports 2019;8(1):31–42.

21. Shimbo D, Barrett Bowling C, Levitan EB, et al. Short-term risk of serious fall injuries in older adults initiating and intensifying treatment with antihypertensive medication. Circ Cardiovasc Qual Outcomes 2016;9(3):222–9.

22. National Academies of Sciences, Engineering, and Medicine. Social isolation and loneliness in older adults: opportunities for the health care system. Washington, DC: National Academies Press; 2020.

23. Hashemi A, Vasquez K, Guishard D, et al. Implementing DASH-aligned congregate meals and self-measured blood pressure in two senior centers: an open label study. Nutr Metabol Cardiovasc Dis 2022;32(8):1998–2009.

24. Khoong EC, Commodore-Mensah Y, Lyles CR, et al. Use of self-measured blood pressure monitoring to improve hypertension equity. Curr Hypertens Rep 2022;24(11):599–613.

25. Liyanage-Don N, Fung D, Phillips E, et al. Implementing home blood pressure monitoring into clinical practice. Curr Hypertens Rep 2019;21(2):14.
26. Kronish IM, Kent S, Moise N, et al. Barriers to conducting ambulatory and home blood pressure monitoring during hypertension screening in the United States. J Am Soc Hypertens 2017;11(9):573–80.
27. Derington CG, King JB, Bryant KB, et al. Cost-effectiveness and challenges of implementing intensive blood pressure goals and team-based care. Curr Hypertens Rep 2019;21(12):91.
28. Meador M, Hannan J, Roy D, et al. Accelerating use of self-measured blood pressure monitoring (smbp) through clinical-community care models. J Community Health 2021;46(1):127–38.
29. Bowling CB, Whitson HE, Johnson TM. 2nd. The 5Ts: preliminary development of a framework to support inclusion of older adults in research. J Am Geriatr Soc 2019;67(2):342–6.
30. Bowling CB, Thomas J, Gierisch JM, et al. Research inclusion across the lifespan: a good start, but there is more work to be done. J Gen Intern Med 2023;38(8): 1966–9.
31. Osborn R, Doty MM, Moulds D, et al. Older americans were sicker and faced more financial barriers to health care than counterparts in other countries. Health Aff (Millwood) 2017;36(12):2123–32.
32. Cutilli CC, Bennett IM. Understanding the health literacy of America: results of the national assessment of adult literacy. Orthop Nurs 2009;28(1):27–32, quiz 33-4.
33. Krishnaswami A, Beavers C, Dorsch MP, et al. Gerotechnology for older adults with cardiovascular diseases: JACC state-of-the-art review. J Am Coll Cardiol 2020;76(22):2650–70.
34. Pew Research Center. Tech adoption climbs among older adults. Available at: https://www.pewresearch.org/internet/wp-content/uploads/sites/9/2017/05/PI_2017.05.17_Older-Americans-Tech_FINAL.pdf. [Accessed 29 January 2024].
35. Jackson SL, Ayala C, Tong X, et al. Clinical implementation of self-measured blood pressure monitoring, 2015-2016. Am J Prev Med 2019;56(1):e13–21.
36. Centers for Disease Control and Prevention. Self-measured blood pressure (SMBP) monitoring. 2023. Available at: https://millionhearts.hhs.gov/tools-protocols/tools/smbp.html. [Accessed 5 February 2024].
37. American Medical Association. Blood pressure devices. 2023. Available at: https://www.validatebp.org. [Accessed 5 February 2024].

Optimal Blood Pressure Targets with Age

Mark A. Supiano, MD, AGSF

KEYWORDS

- Age-friendly care • Cognitive impairment • Dementia • Patient-centered
- Clinical guidelines • Randomized clinical trials • Therapeutic nihilism

KEY POINTS

- In the absence of high disease burden or markedly short predicted remaining life expectancy, a systolic blood pressure (SBP) treatment goal below 130 mm Hg is recommended for the majority of older adults.
- Older adults with high cardiovascular disease or brain health risk, likely, derive greater benefit from a more intensive SBP target level.
- An approach encompassing each of the geriatrics Medications, Mentation, Mobility and What Matters (4M) domains provides a good framework to develop an individualized, optimal, patient-centric SBP treatment target.
- What is good for the heart is also good for the brain!

INTRODUCTION

There have been several important updates to the body of evidence available to inform clinicians and patients regarding the optimal blood pressure (BP) target across all ages, inclusive of older adults since the last issue of *Clinics* devoted to Geriatric Hypertension was published in 2009. Given this review's focus on older adults, it is important to state at the outset that it is possible to solely utilize the systolic blood pressure (SBP) to define stages of hypertension, as well as for the target or goal BP. Also, since isolated diastolic hypertension is so uncommon among older patients, one may correctly classify an older patient's hypertension in almost all cases based entirely on the level of their SBP.

The operational definition for an "optimal" SBP target utilized herein is the *"benefit-based SBP treatment goal based on patient age, comorbidities, and cardiovascular and cognitive impairment risk factors."* Appropriately incorporating patient preferences into this risk/benefit framework requires that additional nuances be considered to assess time to benefit and/or time to harm. Within this framework, this review will

Division of Geriatrics, Spencer Fox Eccles School of Medicine, Center on Aging, University of Utah, 30 North Mario Capecchi Drive, 2nd Floor North, Salt Lake City, UT 84112, USA
E-mail address: mark.supiano@utah.edu

Clin Geriatr Med 40 (2024) 585–595
https://doi.org/10.1016/j.cger.2024.04.002
0749-0690/24/© 2024 Elsevier Inc. All rights reserved.

outline the clinical trial evidence (highlighting randomized clinical trials [RCTs] published since 1990), clinical practice guideline recommendations that have incorporated trial evidence over this time period, and recommend an age-friendly, patient-centric approach to develop a benefit-based SBP optimal target for older adults. One last point regarding any SBP promulgated to be optimal is that the cardiovascular disease (CVD) risks doubles for every 20 mm Hg in SBP above 115 mm Hg.[1]

CLINICAL TRIAL EVIDENCE

There were no data to inform optimal BP targets specific to older adults until 1991 when the results from the placebo-controlled clinical trial, "Systolic Hypertension in the Elderly (SHEP)," were published.[2] This landmark trial provided the first evidence that treating what was then categorized as "isolated systolic hypertension"—an SBP in excess of 160 mm Hg—in older adults was both safe and effective. Prior to this publication, a common belief was that a reasonable goal SBP for older adults was as high as 100 plus their chronologic age in years. This was linked to a perception that the older brain required a higher SBP to ensure adequate cerebral perfusion. **Fig. 1** illustrates the evolution in the evidence basis emanating from SHEP and the additional 3 RCTs that in the ensuing 30 years (**Table 1**) have refined the understanding of the optimal SBP target for older adults and how these data have, in parallel, informed a series of clinical guidelines that have dramatically changed this landscape.

Systolic Hypertension in the Elderly Program

The "SHEP" trial began in 1984 with a primary objective to test the ability of antihypertensive drug treatment to reduce the risk of nonfatal and fatal (total) stroke in adults aged 60 years and older with isolated systolic hypertension, that is, an SBP above 160 mm Hg.[2] The trial enrolled 4736 participants with a mean age of 72 years, 57% were women, and who had a mean entry SBP of 170 mm Hg (range, 160–219 mm Hg). Participants were randomized to placebo or stepped care active treatment with low dose thiazide (step 1) or beta-blocker (step 2) to achieve a target SBP of a 20 mm Hg reduction from baseline (if below 180 mm Hg) or less than 160 mm Hg if baseline exceeded 180 mm Hg. Its results provided the first evidence that antihypertensive drug treatment in older patients with isolated systolic hypertension could be safely accomplished in older adults, and that treatment resulted in a significant (36%) reduction in the incidence of fatal and nonfatal stroke.

Hypertension in the Very Elderly Trial

The "Hypertension in the Very Elderly Trial (HYVET)" extended the SHEP age boundary by enrolling only adults aged 80 years and older to address a very similar primary objective.[3] HYVET recruited 3845 participants (mean age 83.6 years, 60% were female individuals, with an average SBP 173 mm Hg) who were randomized to placebo or active treatment consisting of a nonthiazide diuretic and, if required, an angiotensin-converting enzyme (ACE) inhibitor. The treatment target was an SBP below 150 mm Hg. Due to an unexpected 21% reduction in all-cause mortality in the active treatment group, the trial's data safety committee recommended the trial be ended with median follow-up of only 1.8 years. The active treatment group also had a 30% reduction in fatal and nonfatal stroke and a 64% decrease in the rate of congestive heart failure. The distribution of frailty among HYVET subjects determined from a deficit accumulation approach was found to be very similar to that of comparably aged community-based populations. Moreover, both frail and nonfrail HYVET participants benefited from active treatment.[4] Finally, results from an open-label extension study in which

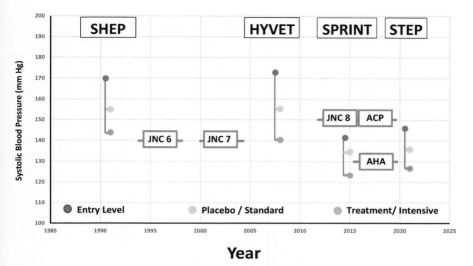

Fig. 1. No RCT data existed prior to 1991 to inform the treatment of what was then referred to as isolated systolic hypertension in older adults. The 4 major RCTs conducted in older adults are depicted in the year of each trial's publication, beginning in 1991 with the Systolic Hypertension in the Elderly Program—SHEP,[2] followed by the Hypertension in the Very Elderly Trial—HYVET,[3] the Systolic Blood Pressure Intervention Trial—SPRINT and SPRINT-Senior,[6,8] and the Strategy of Blood Pressure Intervention in the Elderly Hypertensive Patients trial—STEP.[9] The blue circle and the vertical blue line indicate the average entry SBP levels for each trial and the achieved SBP for the placebo or standard (*yellow circle*) and active or intensive arms (*green circle*). It is important to recognize that the benefits observed with intensive therapy in both SPRINT and STEP are relative to a standard arm whose SBP levels were below the level recommended in guidelines published prior to 2017. The figure's red boxes and the horizontal red lines illustrate the recommended SBP target goal established sequentially over time by the Joint National Committee on the Detection and Prevention of Hypertension's (JNC) 6, 7 and 8 guidelines[1,11,12] and the 2017 guidelines from the American College of Cardiology/AHA Task Force[14] and the ACP and the AAFP.[15] It is noteworthy that there is a significant time lag between the RCT evidence basis and the resulting change in clinical guidelines. The divergent higher 150 mm Hg level promulgated in the JNC 8 and ACP guidelines are discussed in the narrative. (*From* Supiano MA, Williamson JD. New Guidelines and SPRINT Results. Circulation. 2019;140(12):976-978. doi:10.1161/circulatio naha.119.037872.)

placebo subjects switched to active treatment demonstrated that the prior-placebo group achieved the same reduction in stroke by 12 months, suggesting that the time to treatment benefit in this age group is relatively short.[5]

Systolic Blood Pressure Intervention Trial

The "Systolic Blood Pressure Intervention Trial" (SPRINT) and its companion SPRINT "Memory and Cognition in Decreased Hypertension" (MIND) study results—cognitive impairment and brain MRI—were published in 2015 and 2019, respectively.[6,7] After the results from both SHEP and HYVET were published, it was no longer ethically permissible to design a placebo-controlled trial to address the optimal SBP target question. Instead, the SPRINT study design randomized 9361 hypertensive individuals aged 50 years and older without prevalent diabetes but with high cardiovascular disease risk to 1 of 2 SBP targets—usual (<140 mm Hg) or intensive (<120 mm Hg). A

Table 1
Randomized blood pressure lowering clinical trials in older adults

Trial	Publication Year	Enrolled (N)	Age (Mean, years)	Female Individuals (%)	Entry SBP (Mean mm Hg)	Placebo/ Standard SBP (Mean, mm Hg)	Treatment/ Intensive SBP (Mean, mm Hg)	Reduction in Primary Outcome (%)
SHEP	1991	4,736	72.0	57	170.0	155.1	144.0	35% stroke
HYVET	2008	3,845	83.6	60	173.0	155.5	140.5	30% stroke
SPRINT	2015	9,361	67.9	36	139.7	134.6	121.5	25% composite CVD and death
SPRINT Senior	2016	2,636	79.9	38	141.6	134.8	123.4	34% composite CVD and death
STEP	2021	8,511	66.2	53	146.0	135.9	126.7	26% composite CVD and death

Abbreviations: HYVET, Hypertension in the Very Elderly Trial[3]; SHEP, Systolic Hypertension in the Elderly Program[2]; SPRINT, Systolic Blood Pressure Intervention Trial[6]; SPRINT-senior, Intensive vs Standard Blood Pressure Control and Cardiovascular Disease Outcomes in Adults Aged ≥75 y[8]; STEP, Strategy of Blood Pressure Intervention in the Elderly Hypertensive Patients.[9]

subset of 2636 participants aged 75 years and older were recruited into its SPRINT-Senior cohort.[8] Among the older subjects randomized to the intensive arm, there was a significant 34% reduction in the primary composite cardiovascular disease (CVD) outcome and a significant 33% reduction in all-cause mortality at 3.14 years of follow-up when, similar to HYVET, the trial ended early due to its highly positive outcomes (numbers needed to treat 27 and 41, respectively). These results differ neither for the most frail subgroup nor for those with impaired gait speed.

SPRINT MIND was designed to address the hypothesis that the incidence of dementia would be lower with intensive SBP treatment. Although the 17% reduction in adjudicated all-cause probable dementia in the intensive relative to the standard group did not achieve statistical significance, there were significant reductions of the same magnitude in the occurrence of mild cognitive impairment (MCI; 19%; $P = .01$) and in the composite outcome of MCI or dementia (15%; $P = .02$). Longer term cognitive outcome data are currently being obtained in the SPRINT MIND 2020 study to further evaluate the dementia outcome as more cases accrue with extended follow-up. Results are expected by the end of 2024. The companion SPRINT-MRI study provided complementary results demonstrating that intensive therapy was associated with slower progression in the accumulation of white matter hyperintensity volume without significant differences in total brain volume.

Strategy of Blood Pressure Intervention in the Elderly Hypertensive Patients

The "Strategy of Blood Pressure Intervention in the Elderly Hypertensive Patients" (STEP), began in China shortly after SPRINT.[9] A total of 8511 Chinese patients with hypertension (age range 60–80 years) were randomized to an intensive treatment goal (SBP 100 to <130 mm Hg) or a standard goal (130 to <150 mm Hg). In addition to the different racial composition relative to SPRINT, participants in the (STEP) trial were younger (mean age 66.2 years) and in general had lower CVD risk. There were also differences in the measurement protocols, achieved SBP in the 2 arms, and the antihypertensive drug regimens used to achieve the treatment target goals. Nonetheless, similar to SPRINT, the trial ended early, at a follow-up of 3.3 years, when it was evident that its primary CVD outcome was met in favor of the intensive treatment goal. The STEP trial's major conclusion that "a reduction in the systolic blood pressure to less than 130 mm Hg resulted in cardiovascular benefits in older patients with hypertension in China" is largely confirmatory of the SPRINT results. No cognitive outcomes were adjudicated in STEP.

Finally, another RCT conducted in China and quite similar in design to STEP has recently been completed—the "Effects of intensive Systolic blood Pressure lowering treatment in reducing RIsk of vascular evenTs (ESPRIT)" trial.[10] Its preliminary findings were reported in late 2023 are well aligned with the intensive treatment benefits reported in both SPRINT and STEP, but the results have not yet been published.

CLINICAL PRACTICE GUIDELINE RECOMMENDATIONS

Informed by the historical context of these key clinical trials, the parallel evolution of the major clinical practice guidelines will next be discussed with a focus on their recommendations most pertinent to older adults.

Joint National Committee's Sixth Report

Six years after the SHEP trial results were published, the American Heart Association (AHA) Joint National Committee's Sixth Report (JNC 6) was the first guideline to specifically recommend an SBP target for older adults.[11] The "isolated systolic hypertension" classification was effectively sunset in the 1997 JNC 6 guideline when the conjunction linking systolic and diastolic pressures was changed from "and" to "or." Further, hypertension was defined as any SBP in excess of 140 mm Hg. These definitions also emphasize that SBP is a more important CVD risk factor than diastolic BP—especially for individuals aged older than 50 years. Its section devoted to special populations stated, "Treatment of hypertension in older persons has demonstrated major benefits." With regard to a treatment goal, it recommended, "The goal of treatment in older patients should be the same as in younger patients (to <140/90 mm Hg if at all possible), although an interim goal of SBP below 160 mm Hg may be necessary in those patients with marked systolic hypertension."

Joint National Committee's Seventh Report

Very little changed with respect to recommendations for older adults in the Joint National Committee's Seventh Report published in 2003.[1] It stated, "Treatment recommendations for older individuals with hypertension should follow the same principles outlined for the general care of hypertension."

Report from the Panel Members Appointed to the Eighth Joint National Committee

The "Evidence-Based Guideline for the Management of High Blood Pressure in Adults: Report from the Panel Members Appointed to the Eighth Joint National Committee" (also known as JNC 8) recommended a goal BP of less than 150/90 mm Hg for patients between the ages of 60 and 80 years—a deviation from the SBP target level of less than 140 mm Hg that was previously recommended.[12] Significant controversy surrounded this recommendation when it was published in 2014. A dissenting minority opinion from this panel argued for maintaining this goal below 140 mm Hg.[13] Applying benefit-based therapy to adults aged 60 years and older with systolic hypertension who are at high CVD risk is one of the points emphasized by this group in support of their view that the appropriate SBP goal for this group should remain below 140 mm Hg. In addition, the JNC 8 recommendation was at odds with the target goals published in clinical guidelines from many other organizations.

Report of the American College of Cardiology/American Heart Association Task Force on Clinical Practice Guidelines

The 2017 Report of the American College of Cardiology/AHA Task Force "Guideline for the Prevention, Detection, Evaluation, and Management of High Blood Pressure in Adults" marked a departure from the National Heart, Lung, and Blood Institute Joint National Committee structure with its decision to partner with other entities to develop these recommendations.[14] With respect to older adults, this guideline states, "an SBP treatment goal of less than 130 mm Hg is recommended for noninstitutionalized ambulatory community-dwelling adults (≥65 years of age) with an average SBP of 130 mm Hg or higher." The reduction from 140 to 130 mm Hg in the definition of hypertension and, in turn, the optimal SBP recommendation was primarily due to evidence from the SPRINT study. The guideline's second recommendation—"For older adults (≥65 years of age) with hypertension and a high burden of comorbidity and limited life expectancy, clinical judgment, patient preference, and a team-based approach to assess risk/benefit is reasonable for decisions regarding intensity of BP lowering and choice of antihypertensive drugs"—encapsulates the nuances inherent in the complexity of providing care to older persons. Perhaps, especially, among the heterogeneous population of older adults with hypertension, a personalized, patient-centric approach that carefully integrates the individual's risks and benefits of more intensive BP control is necessary. This evaluation should incorporate the patient's additional comorbidities, frailty status, prognosis with regard to projected time to benefit from the intervention, and goals of care.

Clinical Practice Guideline from the American College of Physicians and the American Academy of Family Physicians

Also published in 2017, the "Clinical Practice Guideline from the American College of Physicians (ACP) and the American Academy of Family Physicians (AAFP)" focused on treatment recommendations for adults aged 60 years and older.[15] Notably, these groups recommended a higher SBP target of 150 mm Hg aligning with the 2014 JNC 8 guideline. That said, this recommendation was qualified for those with a history of cerebrovascular disease or at high cardiovascular risk suggesting a target SBP of less than 140 mm Hg for those individuals. These qualifications suggest that there are more similarities than differences between the ACP/AAFP guideline and the ACC/AHA task force guideline. In particular, the ACP/AAFP *conclusion*, "... recommend that clinicians select the treatment goals for adults aged 60 years or older based on a periodic discussion of the benefits and harms of specific blood pressure targets with the patient" aligns quite closely with second recommendation of the ACC/AHA guideline. The challenges inherent in attributing an individual's risks and benefits will be discussed in the final section with a goal to utilize an age-friendly, patient-centric approach to develop a benefit-based SBP optimal target for older adults.

DEVELOPING A PATIENT-CENTRIC, AGE-FRIENDLY APPROACH

The inherent complexity and heterogeneity of older adults with multiple comorbidities that may include cognitive impairment and frailty who also have elevated SBP likely explains why it is challenging to apply a "one size fits all" treat-to-target therapy approach to this population. This leads into the necessity to embrace a patient-centric, age-friendly approach to address an *individual patient's* optimal SBP target.

Age-Friendly Care: the Geriatric 4M Domains

The age-friendly health system initiative was developed to meet a need to more broadly disseminate evidence-based geriatric models of care.[16] A first step in this process was to consolidate this evidence into 4 domains—mobility, medications, mentation, and what matters most—now referred to as the 4 Ms of geriatrics. This framework may be utilized to develop an individualized, patient-centric approach to hypertensive management in older adults.

Mobility

The morbidity and mortality associated with falls in older adults are undeniable. An underlying geriatric medicine principle is that functional status supersedes chronologic age. To that end, a first step in maximizing mobility in older adults is to assess their frailty status and fall risk. A number of frailty assessment tools are available and easily incorporated into clinical care. The NIA Toolkit's Short Performance Physical Battery is one comprehensive example.[17] Its components—usual gait speed and chair stands—may be used independently. Another example is the clinical frailty scale.[18] It bears emphasis that while injurious falls and other adverse events increased with both older age and greater frailty in both HYVET and SPRINT study cohorts, these outcomes were not greater among those randomized to more intensive SBP control.[4,19] In SPRINT, age greater than 75 years was associated with greater risk of syncope, hypotension, and falls, but there was no age-by-treatment interaction for any of the these adverse outcomes.[19] Finally, it should be kept in mind that fall risk is highest in the period of time immediately following initiation or intensification of antihypertensive therapy. Given this, it is important to inform patients of this period of increased risk and to include frequent BP monitoring.

Underlying orthostatic or postural hypotension is a well-recognized fall risk. An important lesson learned from SPRINT was that the prevalence of orthostasis, defined as an SBP less than 110 mm Hg following 1 minute of upright posture, was 10% among patients aged 75 years and older at the screening, baseline visit. This was an exclusion criterion for the trial, and, since patients with this risk factor for falls were not enrolled, the overall tolerance of the intensive 120 mm Hg target was high, even among the oldest and most frail participants.

A final point of relevance to mobility that overlaps with what matters is that 2 common chronic conditions in hypertensive older adults—heart failure and stoke—have a profoundly deleterious impact on mobility functional status. Given that intensive SBP management significantly attenuates the incidence of these 2 outcomes, maintaining mobility will follow.

Medications

Although counterintuitive and contradictory to another tenet of geriatric medicine—avoiding polypharmacy—there is little evidence from any of the clinical trials that the higher number of antihypertensive medications needed to achieve the intensive SBP target was associated with more serious adverse events. Almost all SPRINT participants achieved the 120 mm Hg intensive target on a combination of 3 antihypertensive medication drug classes (an angiotension converting enzyme [ACE] or angiontension receptor blocker [ARB], calcium channel blocker, and a thiazide diuretic, most commonly chlorthalidone). The exception is that higher rates of electrolyte abnormalities were identified in SPRINT, undoubtedly related to thiazide diuretic usage. Additional, counterintuitive, information suggests that there are fewer adverse events with lower doses of multiple antihypertensives than with the formerly espoused stepped care approach wherein maximal dosage of a single antihypertensive was utilized.[20]

Beyond polypharmacy, it is important to ensure that age-appropriate medications and dosages (most often adjusting for renal function) are being prescribed and to minimize exposure to potentially inappropriate medications for older adults.[21] In addition, comprehensive medication reconciliation should also target any medications, including nonsteroidal anti-inflammatory medications and others, that are known to elevate BP.

Mentation

Maintaining cognitive health in older adults with hypertension is another important factor to consider. For this reason, the primary outcome in SHEP, and one that is reported in the other trials, was the reduction in stroke rates in the actively treated participants. Today, there is no question that more intensive SBP control is associated with a significant reduction in the incident stroke rate. Moreover, a meta-analysis of stroke outcomes, which included the 4 RCTs cited earlier, identified that the time to benefit for stroke prevention is rather brief. The study's findings suggested, "200 adults aged ≥65 years would need to be treated for 1.7 years to avoid 1 stroke."[22] Since this is the average remaining life expectancy for a 106 year old woman, these results suggest that almost all older adults with hypertension would benefit with respect to stroke prevention from more intensive treatment.

The potential beneficial effect of intensive SBP control in older adults to maintain cognitive function was not known prior to the SPRINT study results being published. The SPRINT MIND study was the first evidence that the outcomes for adjudicated MCI and the composite of MCI and all-cause dementia were significantly reduced among participants randomized to the intensive SBP target arm. Several subsequent secondary analyses from SPRINT MIND have provided additional important insights: (1) greater cognitive benefit was identified in participants who had the highest baseline risk for cognitive decline[23] and (2) greater time spent in therapeutic BP target range of 110 to 130 mm Hg in the first 3 months postrandomization was associated with lower rates for subsequent dementia.[24,25] More details of the intersection between BP control and brain health are provided in Littig and colleagues.[26]

What Matters Most

Balancing the overall risk–benefit equation across these 3 domains in a patient-centric matter aligns with both "what matters" and the art of medicine. It also aligns with nuances included in the AHA 2017 guideline's second recommendation, "*For older adults with a high burden of comorbidity and limited life expectancy, clinical judgment, patient preference, and a team-based approach to assess risk/benefit is reasonable for decisions regarding intensity of BP lowering and choice of antihypertensive drugs.*"[2] Eliciting what matters most to older adults with hypertension needs to be factored into their ultimate, individualized optimal SBP target. It is important that clinicians fully inform patients of the inherent risks and benefits of managing their hypertension to ensure that a given target SBP level aligns with the patient's preferences. One component of this conversation is an attempt to frame the cardiovascular and cognitive function benefits that are evident with more intensive SBP control in the context of the patient's other competing risks from other chronic conditions. For example, a patient who is at high risk to develop cognitive impairment and for whom preventing dementia matter most, may opt to attempt a more intensive, less than 120 mm Hg, SBP target goal. In other patients with risks that conspire to limit their remaining life expectancy, their time to benefit to achieve the benefits from more intensive SBP control may not be realized and a less-aggressive target may be appropriate. Moreover, especially in the setting of severe baseline cognitive impairment and dementia or functional loss and frailty, the BP-lowering benefits may be neither achievable nor indicated.

FUTURE CONSIDERATIONS

First, of note, neither of the 2017 guidelines incorporated the subsequently published SPRINT MIND evidence that more intensive (an SBP target of 120 mm Hg) target led to a significant reduction in the incidence of MCI. The 2024 AHA/ACC guideline update is currently being developed. Second, there is compelling evidence that ageism contributes to therapeutic nihilism and the reticence of some clinicians to escalate antihypertensive therapy in older adults to achieve their optimal SBP.[27,28] Third, BP control rates are low across all age groups and lowest in older adults. Advances in implementation science are needed to help improve these control rates. Fourth, greater public awareness of new information that is altering (lowering) the SBP range considered to be optimal is needed, including the cognitive benefits inherent with a lower SBP.

CLINICS CARE POINTS

- The operational definition for an "optimal" systolic blood pressure target is the "benefit-based SBP treatment goal based on patient age, comorbidities, and cardiovascular and cognitive impairment risk factors."

- Outcome data from recent randomized clinical trials with respect to mortality, CVD and cognitive benefits support a SBP goal below 130 mm Hg for most older adults.
- The heterogeneity of older adults with multiple comorbidities requires a patient-centric, age-friendly approach to address an individual patient's SBP target goal.

DISCLOSURE

The author discloses funding from the National Institutes of Health and royalties from McGraw-Hill Publishing.

REFERENCES

1. Chobanian AV, Bakris GL, Black HR, et al. The seventh report of the joint national committee on prevention, detection, evaluation, and treatment of high blood pressure: the JNC 7 report. JAMA 2003;289(19):2560–72.
2. SHEP Cooperative Research Group. Prevention of stroke by antihypertensive drug treatment in older persons with isolated systolic hypertension: final results of the systolic hypertension in the elderly program (SHEP). JAMA 1991;265: 3255–64.
3. Beckett NS, Peters R, Fletcher AE, et al. Treatment of hypertension in patients 80 years of age or older. N Engl J Med 2008;358(18):1887–98.
4. Warwick J, Falaschetti E, Rockwood K, et al. No evidence that frailty modifies the positive impact of antihypertensive treatment in very elderly people: an investigation of the impact of frailty upon treatment effect in the HYpertension in the Very Elderly Trial (HYVET) study, a double-blind, placebo-controlled study of antihypertensives in people with hypertension aged 80 and over. BMC Med 2015; 13:78.
5. Beckett N, Peters R, Tuomilehto J, et al. Immediate and late benefits of treating very elderly people with hypertension: results from active treatment extension to Hypertension in the Very Elderly randomised controlled trial. BMJ 2012;344: d7541.
6. Wright JT Jr, Williamson JD, Whelton PK, et al. A randomized trial of intensive versus standard blood-pressure control. N Engl J Med 2015;373(22):2103–16.
7. Nasrallah IM, Pajewski NM, Auchus AP, et al. Association of intensive vs standard blood pressure control with cerebral white matter lesions. JAMA 2019;322(6):524.
8. Williamson JD, Supiano MA, Applegate WB, et al. Intensive vs standard blood pressure control and cardiovascular disease outcomes in adults aged >/=75 years: a randomized clinical trial. JAMA 2016;315(24):2673–82.
9. Zhang W, Zhang S, Deng Y, et al. Trial of intensive blood-pressure control in older patients with hypertension. N Engl J Med 2021;385(14):1268–79.
10. Liu J, Wang B, Li Y, et al. Rationale and design of the effects of intensive systolic blood pressure lowering treatment in reducing risk of vascular evenTs (ESPRIT): a multicenter open-label randomized controlled trial. Am Heart J 2023;257:93–102.
11. Sheps S. The sixth report of the joint national committee on prevention, detection, evaluation, and treatment of high blood pressure. Arch Intern Med 1997;157(21): 2413.
12. James PA, Oparil S, Carter BL, et al. 2014 evidence-based guideline for the management of high blood pressure in adults: report from the panel members appointed to the Eighth Joint National Committee (JNC 8). JAMA 2014;311(5): 507–20.

13. Wright JT Jr, Fine LJ, Lackland DT, et al. Evidence supporting a systolic blood pressure goal of less than 150 mm Hg in patients aged 60 years or older: the minority view. Ann Intern Med 2014;160(7):499–503.
14. Whelton PK, Carey RM, Aronow WS, et al. 2017 ACC/AHA/AAPA/ABC/ACPM/AGS/APhA/ASH/ASPC/NMA/PCNA Guideline for the prevention, detection, evaluation, and management of high blood pressure in adults: a report of the american college of cardiology/american heart association task force on clinical practice guidelines. Circulation 2018;138(17):e484–594.
15. Amir Q, Rich R, Humphrey LL, Frost J, Ann M, Forciea MA, Clinical Guidelines Committee of the American College of Physicians and the Commission on Health of the Public and Science of the American Academy of Family Physicians, Fitterman N, Barry MJ, Horwitch CA, Iorio A, McLean RM. Forciea pharmacologic treatment of hypertension in adults aged 60 years or older to higher versus lower blood pressure targets: a clinical practice guideline from the american college of physicians and the american academy of family physicians. Ann Intern Med 2017;166(6):430–7.
16. Mate K, Fulmer T, Pelton L, et al. Evidence for the 4Ms: Interactions and outcomes across the care continuum. J Aging Health 2021;33(7–8):469–81.
17. De Fátima Ribeiro Silva C, Ohara DG, Matos AP, et al. Short physical performance battery as a measure of physical performance and mortality predictor in older adults: a comprehensive literature review. Int J Environ Res Publ Health 2021;18(20):10612.
18. Rockwood K, Song X, MacKnight C, et al. A global clinical measure of fitness and frailty in elderly people. Can Med Assoc J 2005;173(5):489–95.
19. Sink KM, Evans GW, Shorr RI, et al. Syncope, hypotension, and falls in the treatment of hypertension: results from the randomized clinical systolic blood pressure intervention trial. J Am Geriatr Soc 2018;66(4):679–86.
20. Muñoz D, Uzoije P, Reynolds C, et al. Polypill for cardiovascular disease prevention in an underserved population. N Engl J Med 2019;381(12):1114–23.
21. By the American Geriatrics Society Beers Criteria® Update Expert P. American Geriatrics Society 2023 updated AGS Beers Criteria® for potentially inappropriate medication use in older adults. J Am Geriatr Soc 2023;71(7):2052–81.
22. Ho VS, Cenzer IS, Nguyen BT, et al. Time to benefit for stroke reduction after blood pressure treatment in older adults: a meta-analysis. J Am Geriatr Soc 2022. https://doi.org/10.1111/jgs.17684.
23. Ghazi L, Shen J, Supiano M, et al. Identifying patients for intensive blood pressure treatment based on cognitive benefit a secondary analysis of the sprint randomized clinical trial. JAMA Netw Open 2023;6(5). https://doi.org/10.1001/jamanetworkopen.2023.14443.
24. Huang X, Deng S, Xie W, et al. Time in target range of systolic blood pressure and cognitive outcomes in patients with hypertension. J Am Geriatr Soc 2023. https://doi.org/10.1111/jgs.18641.
25. Li S, Jiang C, Wang Y, et al. Systolic blood pressure time in target range and cognitive outcomes: insights from the SPRINT MIND trial. Hypertension 2023; 80(8):1628–36.
26.. Littig L, Sheth KN, Brickman A, et al. Cognitive function and blood pressure in older adults. Clin Geriatr Med 2024;40(4).
27. Zheutlin AR, Addo DK, Jacobs JA, et al. Evidence for age bias contributing to therapeutic inertia in blood pressure management: a secondary analysis of SPRINT. Hypertension 2023. https://doi.org/10.1161/hypertensionaha.123.21323.
28. Supiano MA, Williamson JD. New guidelines and SPRINT results: Implications for geriatric hypertension. Circulation 2019;140(12):976–8.

Blood Pressure and Cognitive Function in Older Adults

Lauren Littig, BA[a], Kevin N. Sheth, MD[a,b],
Adam M. Brickman, PhD[c], Eva A. Mistry, MBBS, MSCI[d],
Adam de Havenon, MD, MS[a,b],*

KEYWORDS

- Blood pressure • Hypertension • Aging • Cognition • Dementia • Prevention
- Treatment

KEY POINTS

- The relationship between blood pressure and cognitive function is complex and varies across different stages of life. Overall, elevated midlife blood pressure has the strongest association with late-life cognitive decline and dementia, supporting the need for a life course approach to detect and manage hypertension in clinical practice.
- In addition to hypertension, several lines of research suggest additional hemodynamic metrics may synergistically impair cognitive function and increase the risk of dementia. In particular, elevated blood pressure variability, abnormal blood pressure dipping patterns, and markers of vascular stiffness are linked to subsequent cognitive decline and an increased risk of developing incident dementia.
- The association between late-life hypertension control and cognition is less consistent, perhaps reflecting the passing of a critical period of intervention.

INTRODUCTION

Between 2000 and 2050, the global life expectancy at birth is expected to rise from 66 to 77, with the percentage of the population over the age of 65 years projected to rise

Sources of funding: Dr A. de Havenon reports NIH, United States/NINDS funding (K23NS105924, UG3NS130228, R01NS130189). Dr K.N. Sheth by NIH/NINDS (U01NS106513, R01NS110721, R01NR018335, R01EB301114, R01MD016178, U24NS107215, U24NS107136, U24NS129500) and American Heart Association Bugher Award.
[a] Department of Neurology, Yale University, 15 York Street, New Haven, CT 06510, USA;
[b] Center for Brain and Mind Health, Yale University, 15 York Street, New Haven, CT 06510, USA;
[c] Department of Neurology, Columbia University Medical Center, 710 West 168 Street, New York, NY 10032, USA; [d] Department of Neurology and Rehabilitation Medicine, University of Cincinnati, 260 Stetson Street, Cincinnati, OH 45267, USA
* Corresponding author. Department of Neurology, Yale University, 15 York Street, New Haven, CT 06510.
E-mail address: adam.dehavenon@yale.edu

from 7% to 16%.[1] This demographic shift poses an unprecedented challenge to the health care profession, necessitating an improved understanding of the health complications that accompany advancing age. Elevated arterial blood pressure (BP), or hypertension, affects an estimated 1.28 billion adults[2] and over two-thirds of adults aged over 65 years[3] and has been linked to cognitive decline and dementia.[4] Specifically, hypertension is recognized as the primary risk factor for vascular cognitive impairment and dementia (VCID) but is also associated with Alzheimer's disease (AD) dementia.[5] Dementia has a substantial global burden, affecting around 60 million individuals in 2023 with a projected 3 fold increase by 2050.[6] In the United States and other Western countries, the incidence of dementia appears to be declining, but given the rapidly aging population, its prevalence is actually increasing. A growing body of evidence supports hypertension as one of dementia's leading treatable risk factors, which could theoretically prevent or delay up to 20% of dementia cases.[7,8]

Hypertension is often underdiagnosed and poorly controlled, earning it the label of "silent killer" due to its subtle onset usually without overt clinical symptoms.[9] In fact, the World Health Organization estimates that 46% of adults with hypertension are unaware they even have the condition.[2] This underscores the importance of early hypertension detection and management, which if implemented effectively, may mitigate the deleterious effects across the life span and holds promise for alleviating the burden of the anticipated dementia epidemic. This review will consolidate the latest evidence on the relationship between hypertension and cognitive function, offering guidance for clinical practice and emphasizing the importance of early detection and management of hypertension to support brain health in the rapidly aging population.

OBSERVATIONAL RELATIONSHIP BETWEEN BLOOD PRESSURE AND COGNITION

The relationship between BP and cognitive function is complex and varies across different stages of life. Overwhelmingly, research has linked cumulative high BP exposure over the life span to an increased risk of dementia.[10] While this association is strongest for systolic blood pressure (SBP), it also holds true for diastolic blood pressure (DBP).[11] Midlife hypertension has the strongest association with later-life cognitive decline, but associations between elevated SBP in young adulthood, even below standard hypertension thresholds, and midlife cognitive decline have also been identified.[12–14] A nationwide cohort study of Swedish men further reinforces the concept of a cumulative accumulation of dementia risk from hypertension at any life stage, identifying that high SBP in adolescence is a risk factor for the subsequent development of dementia.[15]

A nationwide study of 4.5 million adults aged 60+ years found that the link between BP and dementia risk varies by dementia subtype. While the risk of overall dementia and AD showed a U-shaped association with SBP, with both high (SBP $\geq$160 mm Hg, for overall dementia, hazard ratio [HR] = 1.05, 95% confidence interval [CI] = 1.04–1.07; for AD, HR = 1.03, 95% CI = 1.01–1.05) and low (SBP <100 mm Hg, for overall dementia, HR = 1.13, 95% CI = 1.10–1.17; for AD, HR = 1.17, 95% CI = 1.13–1.22) levels having a significantly higher risk, the risk of probable vascular dementia (VaD) increased linearly with SBP levels (SBP <100 mm Hg, HR = 0.91, 95% CI = 0.83–1.01; SBP $\geq$160 mm Hg, HR = 1.23, 95% CI = 1.17–1.28).[16] All of these associations, however, are attenuated with increasing age.

In older adults, low BP has emerged as a risk factor for poor cognitive performance and even the development of dementia.[11,17–21] Some evidence suggests that higher BP may result in improved cognitive testing results, perhaps reflecting improved cerebral perfusion.[22] However, the relationship is confounded by other medical comorbidities and the high prevalence of antihypertensive treatment by later life as well as residual confounding inherent in these observational studies. Taking those factors into account, numerous studies provide strong evidence that untreated hypertension in later life also contributes to dementia risk and progression.[23–25] Overall, the observational evidence is consistent that hypertension at any age is a risk factor for the development and progression of cognitive impairment.

MECHANISM OF HYPERTENSION'S ASSOCIATION WITH DEMENTIA

Hypertension places stress on blood vessels throughout the body and brain, resulting in damage that leads to neuronal injury or death through numerous diverse mechanisms (**Fig. 1**). Prolonged hypertension can lead to decreased cerebral perfusion

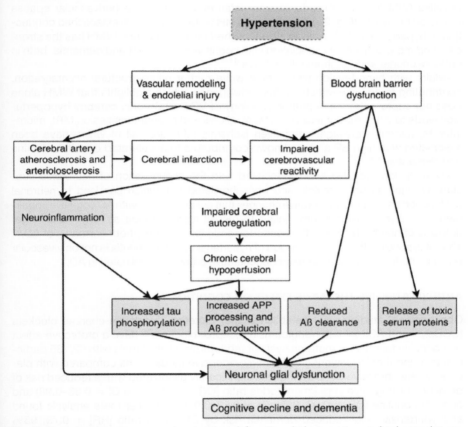

Fig. 1. Hypertension can cause structural and functional changes to cerebral vasculature, leading to impaired cerebral autoregulation, cerebral hypoperfusion, and cerebrovascular disease, such as lacunar infarctions and microhemorrhages. It can also promote neuroinflammation and Alzheimer's-specific pathophysiological processes, including tau phosphorylation and Aβ synthesis and oligomerization, each of which is known to cause neuronal and glial dysfunction and can lead to neurodegeneration and cognitive decline. Aβ, beta-amyloid; APP, amyloid precursor protein. (*From* Walker KA, Gottesman RF. The role of blood pressure and hypertension in dementia. In: Martin CR, Preedy VR, eds. *Diagnosis and Management in Dementia.* Academic Press; 2020:111-126. https://doi.org/10.1016/B978-0-12-815854-8.00008-2; with permission.)

caused by the proliferation of vascular smooth muscle cells, basal lamina alterations, endothelial hyalinosis, fibrosis, and, ultimately, luminal narrowing or vascular occlusion.[26–28] Moreover, it promotes the formation of free radicals and reactive oxygen species (ROS), which leads to cell apoptosis and breakdown of the blood–brain barrier (BBB).[29,30] Fluctuations in BP also induce stress on the vascular wall, affecting endothelial function,[31] and have been associated with cognitive deterioration and cerebrovascular pathology.[32] The association of episodic reduced cerebral perfusion and poorer cognitive test performance further reinforces this connection.[33–35]

The reduction in cerebral blood flow (CBF) secondary to chronic hypertension contributes to the neurodegenerative brain changes linked to hypertension. There is strong support that hypertension may lead to cognitive impairment through the occurrence of cerebral small vessel disease (CSVD),[36] evidenced by white matter hyperintensities (WMHs), microbleeds, lacunar infarcts, and enlarged perivascular spaces visible on brain MRI (**Fig. 2**). In particular, WMH on MRI has a well-established connection to hypertension.[37–40] Among all established MRI biomarkers, WMH has the strongest and most consistent association with cognitive impairment and dementia, both in cross-sectional and longitudinal analyses.[41–45]

Adults with hypertension also exhibit white matter microstructural disintegration, contributing to adverse effects on fluid intelligence, which highlights that WMH alone does not capture the entire pathophysiology of VCID.[46] Chronic cerebral hypoperfusion leads to white matter lesions (WMLs), gliosis and hyperintensities on MRI, microinfarcts, microhemorrhages, and even ischemic infarction, all of which have been associated with high BP and are known contributors to accelerated cognitive decline and dementia.[14,47–51]

Hypertension has also been associated with the accumulation of neurotoxic substances, such as beta-amyloid and phosphorylated tau, which can lead to neuronal dysfunction and neurodegenerative changes that are associated with AD cognitive impairment.[52–54] Hypertension is also linked to medial temporal lobe atrophy[55] and larger amounts of neuritic plaque in the neocortex and hippocampus, both hallmarks of AD.[56] Thus, it is possible that the association of hypertension with dementia is not only vascular but also mediated through the neurodegenerative pathways implicated in AD.

ANTIHYPERTENSIVE THERAPY'S EFFECT ON COGNITION

Observational studies have established that diuretics,[57] calcium-channel blockers (CCBs),[58] and ACE inhibitor/angiotensin receptor blockers[59] have a protective effect on cognitive function. A meta-analysis of randomized clinical trials with 92,135 participants found that BP lowering with antihypertensive medications compared with placebo or less-intensive BP lowering was significantly associated with a reduced risk of dementia or cognitive impairment (odds ratio [OR] = 0.93, 95% CI = 0.88–0.98) and cognitive decline (OR = 0.93, 95% CI = 0.88–0.99).[60] Another meta-analysis found antihypertensive use reduced dementia risk by 21% (risk ratio [RR] = 0.79, 95% CI = 0.70–0.89, I^2 = 68%).[11] However, these results are subject to unmeasured confounding given the heterogeneity of the trial cohorts, the interventions, the length of follow-up, and adjudication of cognitive outcomes.

Multiple trials have found no significant difference in cognitive outcomes between participants on active antihypertensive treatment versus control groups,[61–65] including Systolic Hypertension in the Elderly Program (SHEP), Hypertension in the Very Elderly Trial (HYVET), Heart Outcomes Prevention Evaluation-3 (HOPE-3) trial, and Study on Cognition and Prognosis in the Elderly (SCOPE). The Systolic Hypertension in Europe (Syst-Eur) trial study in the 1990s found that long-term antihypertensive treatment with

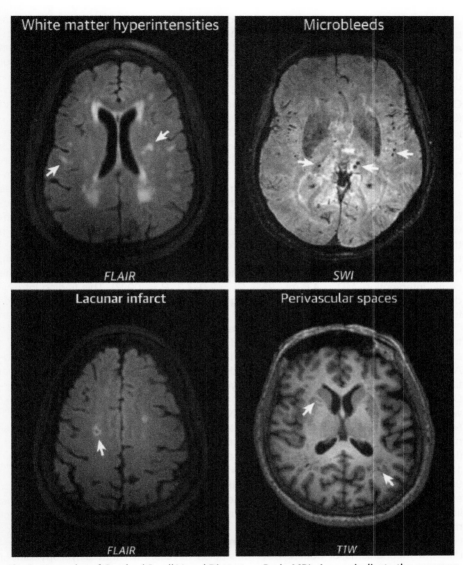

Fig. 2. Examples of Cerebral Small Vessel Disease on Brain MRI. *Arrows* indicate the presence of white matter hyperintensities, microbleeds, lacunar infarcts, and perivascular spaces. FLAIR, fluid attenuation inversion recovery; SWI, susceptibility-weighted imaging; T1W, T1 weighted. (*From* Amier RP, Marcks N, Hooghiemstra AM, et al. Hypertensive Exposure Markers by MRI in Relation to Cerebral Small Vessel Disease and Cognitive Impairment. JACC: Cardiovascular Imaging. 2021;14(1):176-185. https://doi.org/10.1016/j.jcmg.2020.06. 040; with permission.)

nitrendipine, a dihydropyridine CCB, may reduce dementia risk by 50% (95% CI = 0.0–0.76; P = .05),[66] but had a total of only 33 dementia events in a cohort of 2418 participants followed for 2 years. The resulting imprecision of the effect size precludes definitive interpretation.

The Perindopril Protection Against Recurrent Stroke Study (PROGRESS) trial enrolled a cohort of 6105 participants with prior stroke or transient ischemic attack and found that BP lowering with perindopril and indapamide therapy produced a relative risk reduction of 19% (95% CI = 0.04–0.32; P = .01) for cognitive decline.[67] Additional analyses showed that this effect was due to a reduction in recurrent stroke. However, 2 other trials with a harmonized cohort of over 30,000 participants from Ongoing Telmisartan Alone and in Combination with Ramipril Global End Point Trial (ONTARGET) and Telmisartan Randomized AssessmeNt Study in ACE iNtolerant subjects with cardiovascular Disease (TRANSCEND), including a high proportion of participants with prior stroke, found no benefit of antihypertensive treatment on cognition (95% CI = 0.89–1.06; P = .53 and 95% CI = 0.95–1.27; P = .22, respectively).[68]

Action to Control Cardiovascular Risk in Diabetes MIND (ACCORD-MIND) was a substudy of the ACCORD trial in participants with type 2 diabetes that studied the effects of intensive BP lowering and glycemic control on cognitive function and brain volume.[69] The study found no significant differences in cognitive function between the intensive and standard BP treatment groups (MD = 0.32 for Digit Symbol Substitution Test score, 95% CI = −0.28–0.91; P = .2997), though there was a significantly higher total brain volume on MRI after 40 months in the group receiving intensive glycemic intervention (MD = 4.6 mL, 95% CI = 2.0–7.3; P = .0007). This finding introduces the possibility that structural changes related to hypertension may precede functional changes.

Despite the prior research, there continued to be equipoise because none of these trials conducted a follow-up period exceeding 4 years that also included a thorough expert review of cases involving dementia and mild cognitive impairment (MCI). Attempting to reduce the uncertainty regarding antihypertensive treatment and cognition, the Systolic Blood Pressure Intervention Trial Memory and Cognition in Decreased Hypertension (SPRINT-MIND)[70] ancillary to the SPRINT trial was designed with more rigor and longer follow-up. SPRINT-MIND found that intensive SBP control (<120 mm Hg; n = 4278) compared with a standard SBP treatment goal (<140 mm Hg; n = 4385) in patients with hypertension significantly reduced the risk of MCI by 19% (HR = 0.81, 95% CI = 0.70–0.95, P = .01) and combined MCI/probable dementia by 15% (HR = 0.85, 95% CI = 0.74–0.97, P=.02), but not dementia alone (HR = 0.83, 95% CI = 0.67–1.04, P = .10). Importantly, there were no clinically meaningful adverse effects of intensive SBP control in older patients, those with low baseline DBP, borderline kidney disease, or other pertinent subgroups. The results of the trials are summarized in **Table 1**.

Not all antihypertensives have neuroprotective properties, as they each have different mechanisms of action. Several studies have shown that dihydropyridine CCBs do have neuroprotective effects,[66,71–75] attributed to their high lipophilicity and ability to cross the BBB to regulate intracellular calcium levels. High intracellular calcium levels lead to vasoconstriction, reducing CBF, and have been associated with increased production of β-amyloid peptide,[76] ROS,[77] and tau accumulation,[78] all of which are linked to the development of AD and VaD. Dihydropyridines and CCBs, in general, work by blocking L-type voltage-gated calcium channels (L-VGCCs) to prevent high levels of intracellular calcium, thus mitigating its role in the pathogenesis of AD and VaD. This mechanism is illustrated in **Fig. 3**.

Several interesting substudies analyzing brain MRI at baseline and follow-up have emerged out of the SPRINT-MIND trial. One substudy showed that intensive BP treatment, compared with standard treatment, was associated with a smaller increase of WMLs (644.5 vs 1258.1 mm^3), a smaller decrease in fractional anisotropy (mean

Table 1
Characteristics of the selected randomized clinical trials examining the effect of antihypertensive therapy on cognition

Study	Total N (Treatment Group)	Age (SD) at Baseline	Follow-up (years)	Intervention/Antihypertensive Agents Studied	Outcome of Interest	Effects of Treatment
SHEP[64]	N = 4608 (2317)	74	5	Diuretic and β-blocker vs placebo	Cognition	No effect
HYVET[62]	N = 3336 (1687)	84 (3)	2.2	Diuretic and ACE inhibitor vs placebo	Dementia	No effect
HOPE-3[65]	N = 1626 (Candesartan/HCTZ = 405, rosuvastatin = 401, Combination = 406)	74 (3.5)	5.7	Candesartan/hydrochlorothiazide, rosuvastatin, or their combination vs placebo	Cognition	No effect
SCOPE[61]	N = 4964 (2477)	76	4	ARB vs placebo	Cognition and dementia	No effect
Syst-Eur[59]	N = 2418 (1238)	70 (7)	2	CCB ± diuretic vs placebo	Dementia	Protective
PROGRESS[67]	N = 6105 (3054)	64 (10)	4	ACE inhibitor ± diuretic vs placebo	Cognition and dementia	Protective for patients with recurrent stroke
ONTARGET[68]	N = 25,620 (ARB = 8542, ACE inhibitor = 8576, combination = 8502)	66 (7)	4.6	ACE inhibitor, ARB, or their combination vs placebo	Cognition	No effect
TRANSCEND[68]	N = 5231 (2972)	67 (7)	4.7	ARB vs placebo	Cognition and dementia	No effect
ACCORD-MIND[95]	N = 2977 (1358)	62 (6)	3.3	Intensive glycemic treatment (HbA1c <6%) vs standard (HbA1c 7%–7.9%) and intensive BP treatment (<120 mm Hg) vs standard (<140 mm Hg)	Cognition	No effect
SPRINT-MIND[70]	N = 9361 (4678)	68	3.3	Intensive BP treatment (<120 mm Hg) vs standard treatment (<140 mm Hg)	MCI and dementia	Intensive BP treatment was protective against MCI and MCI/dementia combined

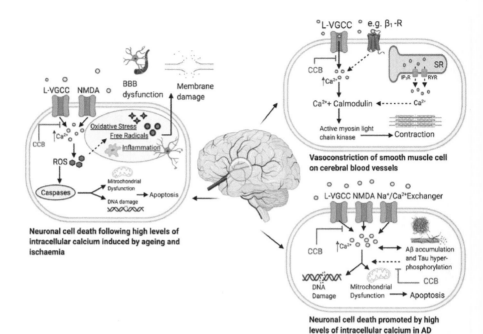

Fig. 3. Role of intracellular calcium in the pathogenesis of AD and VaD, illustrating the potential neuroprotective effect of CCBs. Aβ, amyloid-β; AD, Alzheimer's disease; β1-R, beta1-adrenoceptor; BBB, blood–brain barrier; CCB, calcium channel blocker; IP3R, 1,4,5-triphosphate receptor; L-VGCC, L-type voltage-gated calcium channel; NDMA, N-methyl-d-aspartate; ROS, reactive oxygen species; RYR, ryanodine receptor; SR, sarcoplasmic reticulum. (Created with BioRender.com.)

change, -0.0026 vs -0.0062 for deep white matter [DWM] regions and -0.0011 vs -0.0040 for superficially located white mattter (SWM) regions), a smaller increase in mean diffusivity (0.0044 vs 0.0184 for DWM regions and 0.0038 vs 0.0073 for SWM regions), and a larger increase in CBF (4.6 mL/100 mg/min vs 3.7 mL/100 mg/min).[79] Another interesting substudy in SPRINT-MIND found that at 48 months follow-up, in the intensive BP control arm, WMH volume increased by 0.28 versus a larger increase of 0.92 mL in the standard BP control arm (*P* = .004).[80] A similar result was also found in an analysis of 314 participants in the ACCORD-MIND trial, where those in the intensive BP control arm had a WMH increase of 0.67 versus 1.16 mL in the control arm (*P* = .001).[81] Similar results were found in a small trial of older participants with established CSVD.[82] Finally, an analysis of MRI data from SPRINT in combination with INFINITY (Intensive vs Standard Blood Pressure Lowering to Prevent Functional Decline in Older People) found that intensive SBP control was associated with less WMH progression than the standard SBP treatment (0.29 vs 0.48 mL, *P* = .03).[83] The relative consistency of this finding across different clinical trials shows that a putative benefit of hypertension control on cognition could be mediated through a reduction of WMH progression, in addition to reducing stroke risk.

OTHER BLOOD PRESSURE METRICS AND MEASUREMENT METHODS

New BP metrics and monitoring methods have provided valuable insights into the relationship of other BP-related factors with cognition, offering a more comprehensive understanding of this relationship. Blood pressure variability (BPV) reflects fluctuations in BP over distinct time scales, encompassing very short-term to long-term variations. Higher BPV has emerged as an indicator of impaired cardiovascular regulation, correlating with adverse outcomes such as stroke, coronary artery disease, heart failure, end-stage renal disease, and dementia incidence.[32]

The Three-City Study found a significant association between a higher BPV and an increased risk of incident dementia. In this community-based older adult cohort, participants in the highest decile of BPV over the 8 year follow-up period had a 77% increased risk of dementia compared with those in the lowest decile (P = .007).[84] Work with the S.AGES cohort (Sujets AGES—Aged Subjects) linked higher visit-to-visit BPV to poorer cognitive function and greater risk of dementia, independent of baseline BP levels (1-SD increase of systolic BPV: HR = 1.23, 95% CI = 1.01–1.50, P = .04), with similar results reported for diastolic BPV (P < .01).[47] Substantiating this, the Coronary Artery Risk Development in Young Adults (CARDIA) study[85] demonstrated that elevated long-term systolic and diastolic BPV, independent of hypertension, in young adulthood are linked to worse midlife psychomotor speed (β standard error [SE]: −0.025 [0.006] and −0.029 [0.007], respectively; P<.001) and poorer performance on verbal memory tests (β [SE]: −0.016 [0.006] and −0.021 [0.007], respectively; P<.05). An analysis of data from the Atherosclerosis Risk in Communities study supports these findings, also associating greater visit-to-visit BPV during midlife with lower cognitive function over 25 years of follow-up.[86]

A post hoc analysis of the SPRINT-MIND trial found that the rate of dementia increased by ascending BPV tertile, even in cases with excellent BP control.[87] In the SPRINT-MIND cohort, compared to the lowest tertile of BPV, the highest tertile of BPV increased the risk of dementia in both unadjusted (HR = 2.36, 95% CI = 1.77–3.15) and adjusted (HR = 1.69, 95% CI = 1.25–2.28) models. They also found that the highest tertile of BPV was associated with both MCI (adjusted HR = 1.40, 95% CI = 1.14–1.71) and the composite of dementia/MCI (adjusted HR = 1.43, 95% CI = 1.20–1.71). A meta-analysis of studies found dementia and cognitive impairment to be associated with higher systolic BPV (OR = 1.25, 95% CI = 1.16–1.35), mean systolic pressure (OR = 1.12, 95% CI = 1.02–1.29), DBPV (OR = 1.20, 95% CI = 1.12–1.29), and mean diastolic pressure (OR = 1.16, 95% CI = 1.04–1.29). Further, they found that the BPV effect size was stronger than the mean BP effect size on dementia or cognitive impairment.[88] However, these are all secondary and post hoc analyses. Additional research is needed to understand how to reduce BPV and to determine if its reduction lowers the risk of cognitive impairment or dementia.

In addition to BPV, pulse pressure (PP) and pulse wave velocity (PWV) are highly correlated with cognitive decline. Elevated levels of PP and PWV have been associated with poorer cognitive test performance[89] and glymphatic dysfunction, a hallmark of AD. Moreover, PP and PWV serve as markers of arterial stiffness,[90] suggesting they may be better indicators of the chronicity of hypertension than hypertension itself (More information is provided in Tuday and colleagues[91]). However, similar to BPV, additional research is needed to determine their potential as a therapeutic target for dementia.[92]

24-hour Ambulatory Blood Pressure Monitoring

24-hour ambulatory BP monitoring (ABPM) is another method of BP monitoring that captures the physiologic variance of BP throughout the day, termed the "circadian BP rhythm." A normal pattern is characterized by fluctuations in a diurnal pattern and a normal 10% to 20% drop in nighttime BP values.[32] Patients can be categorized as "dippers" (≥10%) who exhibit a normal dipping BP pattern, "nondippers" (<10%), and "reverse dippers" (dipping <0%). Longitudinal studies employing 24-hour ABPM reveal that abnormal dipping (less than 10%) precedes cognitive decline, emphasizing the significance of analyzing BP profiles beyond office measurements.

A meta-analysis of studies found dippers to have a 51% (OR = 0.49, 95% CI = 0.35–0.69) lower risk of abnormal cognitive function (composite of cognitive impairment or dementia) and a 63% (OR = 0.37, 95% CI = 0.23–0.61) lower risk of dementia alone, compared to nondippers.[6] Moreover, they found reverse dippers to have a 6 fold higher risk (OR = 6.06, 95% CI = 3.15–11.64) of abnormal cognitive function compared to the normal dippers. Reverse dippers were also found to perform worse in global function neuropsychological tests compared with both normal and nondippers (standardized mean difference [SMD] = −0.66, 95% CI = −0.93 to −0.39).[6] This evidence is in line with studies that found that nondipping and reverse-dipping patterns are associated with WMH, silent cerebral infarcts, and brain atrophy.[93]

RECOMMENDATIONS

Given the strong association between midlife hypertension and late-life cognitive function, a life course approach is necessary in clinical practice to identify individuals who may be at elevated risk of cognitive decline secondary to uncontrolled BP. According to the 2017 American College of Cardiology/American Heart Association Hypertension Clinical Guideline,[94] the standards for accurate BP measurements are as follows:

- Normal: <120/<80 mm Hg
- Elevated: 120 to 129/<80 mm Hg
- Stage 1 Hypertension: 130 to 139 or 80 to 89 mm Hg
- Stage 2 Hypertension: ≥140 or ≥90 mm Hg

This guideline recommends that the diagnosis of hypertension should be confirmed with out-of-office self-monitoring of BP, such as home or 24-hour ABPM, which affords clinicians a more complete picture of one's BP profile and can tailor intervention at the individual level. Based on the cognitive results of SPRINT-MIND and the overall cardiovascular and mortality benefits of intensive SBP reduction to less than 120 mm Hg,[10,95–98] it is reasonable to recommend that patients with stage 1 or stage 2 hypertension receive antihypertensive medication to target a goal of less than 120/80 mm Hg, especially those at high risk for cognitive decline and dementia. In patients with elevated BP but not overt hypertension, a more conservative approach focusing on diet, exercise, and other nonmedication therapies seems to be reasonable. However, if that approach fails, initiation of antihypertensive medication should also be considered.

SUMMARY

This review underscores the critical role of hypertension management across the life span in reducing the risk of cognitive decline and dementia. Observational and clinical evidence solidifies the association between hypertension and various forms of cognitive impairment, indicating that effective BP control can serve as a pivotal intervention in preserving cognitive health. Novel metrics and monitoring methods, such as BPV and 24-hour ABPM, offer deeper insights into the complex relationship between hypertension and cognitive function, suggesting more personalized approaches to hypertension management. The findings advocate for a life course approach to BP monitoring and control, emphasizing early detection and intervention. Ultimately, addressing hypertension effectively not only promises to enhance cardiovascular health but also to mitigate the burgeoning global burden of dementia, highlighting the necessity for health care systems to adapt and prioritize hypertension management in clinical practice.

CLINICS CARE POINTS

- While there is no definitive evidence that control of hypertension prevents dementia, there is compelling mechanistic evidence supporting the association between hypertension and Alzheimer's and VCID. This underscores the critical role of hypertension prevention rather than treatment in clinical practice for the preservation of cognitive function.
- Nonetheless, given the benefit in reducing the incidence of MCI seen in SPRINT-MIND and the difficulty of studying this outcome, we recommend aggressive control of hypertension, particularly among younger patients, for the maintenance of cognitive function in later life.
- We recommend at-home BP monitoring and lifestyle modifications in conjunction with antihypertensive therapy as a strategy to personalize care for individuals with hypertension or those at risk for dementia.

DISCLOSURE

Dr A. de Havenon has received consultant fees from Novo Nordisk, royalty fees from UpToDate, and has equity in TitinKM and Certus. Dr K.N. Sheth reports compensation from Sense and Zoll, for data and safety monitoring services; compensation from Cerevasc, CSL Behring, Rhaeos and Astrocyte for consultant services; a patent for Stroke wearables licensed to Alva Health. Dr A.M. Brickman serves as a scientific advisor/consultant to Cognito Therapeutics, Cognition Therapeutics, and CogState. He serves on data safety and monitoring boards for Albert Einstein College of Medicine and University of Illinois. Dr A.M. Brickman has a patent for white matter hyperintensity quantification (patent # 9867566) and a patent pending for microbleed detection (publication #20230298170). Dr E.A. Mistry receives consultant fees from AbbVie and RAPID AI.

REFERENCES

1. World population prospects - population division - united nations. Available at: https://population.un.org/wpp/Graphs/Probabilistic/EX/BothSexes/840. [Accessed 22 December 2023].
2. Hypertension. Available at: https://www.who.int/news-room/fact-sheets/detail/hypertension. [Accessed 28 February 2024].
3. Iadecola C, Yaffe K, Biller J, et al. Impact of hypertension on cognitive function: a scientific statement from the american heart association. Hypertension 2016; 68(6):e67–94.
4. Xu W, Tan L, Wang HF, et al. Meta-analysis of modifiable risk factors for Alzheimer's disease. J Neurol Neurosurg Psychiatry 2015;86(12):1299–306.
5. Barba R, Martínez-Espinosa S, Rodríguez-García E, et al. Poststroke dementia. Stroke 2000;31(7):1494–501.
6. Gavriilaki M, Anyfanti P, Mastrogiannis K, et al. Association between ambulatory blood pressure monitoring patterns with cognitive function and risk of dementia: a systematic review and meta-analysis. Aging Clin Exp Res 2023;35(4):745–61.
7. Livingston G, Huntley J, Sommerlad A, et al. Dementia prevention, intervention, and care: 2020 report of the Lancet Commission. Lancet 2020;396(10248): 413–46.

8. Mulligan MD, Murphy R, Reddin C, et al. Population attributable fraction of hypertension for dementia: global, regional, and national estimates for 186 countries. eClinicalMedicine 2023;60:102012.

9. Research C for DE and. High blood pressure–understanding the silent killer. FDA; 2023. Available at: https://www.fda.gov/drugs/special-features/high-blood-pressure-understanding-silent-killer. [Accessed 15 February 2024].

10. Walker KA, Gottesman RF. Chapter 8 - the role of blood pressure and hypertension in dementia. In: Martin CR, Preedy VR, editors. Diagnosis and management in dementia. Cambridge, MA: Academic Press; 2020. p. 111–26.

11. Ou YN, Tan CC, Shen XN, et al. Blood pressure and risks of cognitive impairment and dementia: a systematic review and meta-analysis of 209 prospective studies. Hypertension 2020;76(1):217–25.

12. Suhr JA, Stewart JC, France CR. The relationship between blood pressure and cognitive performance in the third national health and nutrition examination survey (NHANES III). Psychosom Med 2004;66(3):291.

13. Pavlik VN, Hyman DJ, Doody R. Cardiovascular risk factors and cognitive function in adults 30–59 years of age (NHANES III). Neuroepidemiology 2004; 24(1–2):42–50.

14. Mahinrad S, Kurian S, Garner CR, et al. Cumulative blood pressure exposure during young adulthood and mobility and cognitive function in midlife. Circulation 2020;141(9):712–24.

15. Nordström P, Nordström A, Eriksson M, et al. Risk factors in late adolescence for young-onset dementia in men: a nationwide cohort study. JAMA Intern Med 2013; 173(17):1612–8.

16. Lee CJ, Lee JY, Han K, et al. Blood pressure levels and risks of dementia: a nationwide study of 4.5 million people. Hypertension 2022;79(1):218–29.

17. Kähönen-Väre M, Brunni-Hakala S, Lindroos M, et al. Left ventricular hypertrophy and blood pressure as predictors of cognitive decline in old age. Aging Clin Exp Res 2004;16(2):147–52.

18. Axelsson J, Reinprecht F, Siennicki-Lantz A, et al. Low ambulatory blood pressure is associated with lower cognitive function in healthy elderly men. Blood Pres Monit 2008;13(5):269–75.

19. Knecht S, Wersching H, Lohmann H, et al. How much does hypertension affect cognition?: explained variance in cross-sectional analysis of non-demented community-dwelling individuals in the SEARCH study. J Neurol Sci 2009;283(1–2): 149–52.

20. Nilsson SE, Read S, Berg S, et al. Low systolic blood pressure is associated with impaired cognitive function in the oldest old: longitudinal observations in a population-based sample 80 years and older. Aging Clin Exp Res 2007; 19(1):41–7.

21. Forte G, De Pascalis V, Favieri F, et al. Effects of blood pressure on cognitive performance: a systematic review. J Clin Med 2019;9(1):34.

22. Obisesan TO, Obisesan OA, Martins S, et al. High blood pressure, hypertension, and high pulse pressure are associated with poorer cognitive function in persons aged 60 and older: the Third National Health and Nutrition Examination Survey. J Am Geriatr Soc 2008;56(3):501–9.

23. Levine DA, Galecki AT, Langa KM, et al. Blood pressure and cognitive decline over 8 years in middle-aged and older black and white americans. Hypertension 2019;73(2):310–8.

24. Qiu C, Winblad B, Fratiglioni L. The age-dependent relation of blood pressure to cognitive function and dementia. Lancet Neurol 2005;4(8):487–99.

25. Waldstein SR, Giggey PP, Thayer JF, et al. Nonlinear relations of blood pressure to cognitive function. Hypertension 2005;45(3):374–9.

26. Perlmutter LS, Barrón E, Saperia D, et al. Association between vascular basement membrane components and the lesions of Alzheimer's disease. J Neurosci Res 1991;30(4):673–81.

27. Muela HCS, Costa-Hong VA, Yassuda MS, et al. Higher arterial stiffness is associated with lower cognitive performance in patients with hypertension. J Clin Hypertens (Greenwich) 2018;20(1):22–30.

28. Singer J, Trollor JN, Baune BT, et al. Arterial stiffness, the brain and cognition: a systematic review. Ageing Res Rev 2014;15:16–27.

29. Sagar S, Kallo IJ, Kaul N, et al. Oxygen free radicals in essential hypertension. Mol Cell Biochem 1992;111(1):103–8.

30. Lagrange P, Romero IA, Minn A, et al. Transendothelial permeability changes induced by free radicals in an in vitro model of the blood-brain barrier. Free Radic Biol Med 1999;27(5):667–72.

31. Diaz KM, Veerabhadrappa P, Kashem MA, et al. Visit-to-visit and 24-h blood pressure variability: association with endothelial and smooth muscle function in African Americans. J Hum Hypertens 2013;27(11):671–7.

32. Parati G, Bilo G, Kollias A, et al. Blood pressure variability: methodological aspects, clinical relevance and practical indications for management - a European Society of Hypertension position paper. J Hypertens 2023;41(4):527–44.

33. Tsolaki M, Sakka V, Gerasimou G, et al. Correlation of rCBF (SPECT), CSF tau, and cognitive function in patients with dementia of the Alzheimer's type, other types of dementia, and control subjects. Am J Alzheimers Dis Other Demen 2001;16(1):21–31.

34. Jagust WJ, Eberling JL, Reed BR, et al. Clinical studies of cerebral blood flow in Alzheimer's disease. Ann N Y Acad Sci 1997;826:254–62.

35. Ushijima Y, Okuyama C, Mori S, et al. Relationship between cognitive function and regional cerebral blood flow in Alzheimer's disease. Nucl Med Commun 2002;23(8):779–84.

36. Amier RP, Marcks N, Hooghiemstra AM, et al. Hypertensive exposure markers by MRI in relation to cerebral small vessel disease and cognitive impairment. JACC: Cardiovascular Imaging 2021;14(1):176–85.

37. Bryan RN, Cai J, Burke G, et al. Prevalence and anatomic characteristics of infarct-like lesions on MR images of middle-aged adults: the atherosclerosis risk in communities study. AJNR Am J Neuroradiol 1999;20(7):1273–80.

38. Liao Duanping, Cooper Lawton, Cai Jianwen, et al. Presence and severity of cerebral white matter lesions and hypertension, its treatment, and its control. Stroke 1996;27(12):2262–70.

39. Prabhakaran S, Wright CB, Yoshita M, et al. Prevalence and determinants of subclinical brain infarction: the Northern Manhattan Study. Neurology 2008;70(6):425–30.

40. Poels MMF, Ikram MA, van der Lugt A, et al. Incidence of cerebral microbleeds in the general population: the Rotterdam Scan Study. Stroke 2011;42(3):656–61.

41. Mosley TH, Knopman DS, Catellier DJ, et al. Cerebral MRI findings and cognitive functioning: the Atherosclerosis Risk in Communities study. Neurology 2005;64(12):2056–62.

42. Prins ND, van Dijk EJ, den Heijer T, et al. Cerebral small-vessel disease and decline in information processing speed, executive function and memory. Brain 2005;128(Pt 9):2034–41.

43. de Havenon A, Sheth KN, Yeatts SD, et al. White matter hyperintensity progression is associated with incident probable dementia or mild cognitive impairment. Stroke Vasc Neurol 2022;7(4):364–6.

44. Brickman AM, Provenzano FA, Muraskin J, et al. Regional white matter hyperintensity volume, not hippocampal atrophy, predicts incident Alzheimer's disease in the community. Arch Neurol 2012;69(12):1621–7.

45. Debette S, Schilling S, Duperron MG, et al. Clinical significance of magnetic resonance imaging markers of vascular brain injury: a systematic review and meta-analysis. JAMA Neurol 2019;76(1):81–94.

46. Acosta JN, Haider SP, Rivier C, et al. Blood pressure-related white matter microstructural disintegrity and associated cognitive function impairment in asymptomatic adults. Stroke Vasc Neurol 2023;8(5). https://doi.org/10.1136/svn-2022-001929.

47. Rouch L, Cestac P, Sallerin B, et al. Visit-to-visit blood pressure variability is associated with cognitive decline and incident dementia: the SAGES cohort. Hypertension 2020;76(4):1280–8.

48. Levine DA, Springer MV, Brodtmann A. Blood pressure and vascular cognitive impairment. Stroke 2022;53(4):1104–13.

49. Iadecola C, Gottesman RF. Neurovascular and cognitive dysfunction in hypertension. Circ Res 2019;124(7):1025–44.

50. Pantoni L, Basile AM, Pracucci G, et al. Impact of age-related cerebral white matter changes on the transition to disability – the LADIS study: rationale, design and methodology. Neuroepidemiology 2005;24(1–2):51–62.

51. Verdelho A, Madureira S, Moleiro C, et al. White matter changes and diabetes predict cognitive decline in the elderly: the LADIS study. Neurology 2010;75(2): 160–7.

52. Zlokovic BV. Neurovascular pathways to neurodegeneration in Alzheimer's disease and other disorders. Nat Rev Neurosci 2011;12(12):723–38.

53. Kim T, Yi D, Byun MS, et al. Synergistic interaction of high blood pressure and cerebral beta-amyloid on tau pathology. Alzheimer's Res Ther 2022;14(1):193.

54. Hu H, Meng L, Bi YL, et al. Tau pathologies mediate the association of blood pressure with cognitive impairment in adults without dementia: the CABLE study. Alzheimers Dement 2022;18(1):53–64.

55. Korf ESC, White LR, Scheltens P, et al. Midlife blood pressure and the risk of hippocampal atrophy. Hypertension 2004;44(1):29–34.

56. Obisesan TO. Hypertension and cognitive function. Clin Geriatr Med 2009;25(2): 259–88.

57. Yasar S, Lin FM, Fried LP, et al. Diuretic use is associated with better learning and memory in older adults in the Ginkgo Evaluation of Memory study. Alzheimer's Dementia 2012;8(3):188–95.

58. Hussain S, Singh A, Rahman SO, et al. Calcium channel blocker use reduces incident dementia risk in elderly hypertensive patients: a meta-analysis of prospective studies. Neurosci Lett 2018;671:120–7.

59. Ye R, Hu Y, Yao A, et al. Impact of renin–angiotensin system-targeting antihypertensive drugs on treatment of Alzheimer's disease: a meta-analysis. Int J Clin Pract 2015;69(6):674–81.

60. Hughes D, Judge C, Murphy R, et al. Association of blood pressure lowering with incident dementia or cognitive impairment. JAMA 2020;323(19):1–12.

61. Lithell H, Hansson L, Skoog I, et al. The study on cognition and prognosis in the elderly (SCOPE): principal results of a randomized double-blind intervention trial. J Hypertens 2003;21(5):875–86.

62. Peters R, Beckett N, Forette F, et al. Incident dementia and blood pressure lowering in the Hypertension in the Very Elderly Trial cognitive function assessment (HYVET-COG): a double-blind, placebo controlled trial. Lancet Neurol 2008;7(8):683–9.

63. Gurland BJ, Teresi J, Smith WM, et al. Effects of treatment for isolated systolic hypertension on cognitive status and depression in the elderly. J Am Geriatr Soc 1988;36(11):1015–22.

64. Di Bari M, Pahor M, Franse LV, et al. Dementia and disability outcomes in large hypertension trials: lessons learned from the systolic hypertension in the elderly program (SHEP) trial. Am J Epidemiol 2001;153(1):72–8.

65. Bosch J, O'Donnell M, Swaminathan B, et al. Effects of blood pressure and lipid lowering on cognition. Neurology 2019;92(13):e1435–46.

66. Forette F, Seux ML, Staessen JA, et al. Prevention of dementia in randomised double-blind placebo-controlled Systolic Hypertension in Europe (Syst-Eur) trial. Lancet 1998;352(9137):1347–51.

67. The PROGRESS Collaborative Group*. Effects of blood pressure lowering with perindopril and indapamide therapy on dementia and cognitive decline in patients with cerebrovascular disease. Arch Intern Med 2003;163(9):1069–75.

68. Anderson C, Teo K, Gao P, et al. Renin-angiotensin system blockade and cognitive function in patients at high risk of cardiovascular disease: analysis of data from the ONTARGET and TRANSCEND studies. Lancet Neurol 2011;10(1):43–53.

69. Launer LJ, Miller ME, Williamson JD, et al. Effects of intensive glucose lowering on brain structure and function in people with type 2 diabetes (ACCORD MIND): a randomised open-label substudy. Lancet Neurol 2011;10(11):969–77.

70. Kjeldsen SE, Narkiewicz K, Burnier M, et al. Intensive blood pressure lowering prevents mild cognitive impairment and possible dementia and slows development of white matter lesions in brain: the SPRINT Memory and Cognition IN Decreased Hypertension (SPRINT MIND) study. Blood Pres 2018;27(5):247–8.

71. Levere TE, Walker A. Old age and cognition: enhancement of recent memory in aged rats by the calcium channel blocker nimodipine. Neurobiol Aging 1992;13(1):63–6.

72. Levy A, Kong RM, Stillman MJ, et al. Nimodipine improves spatial working memory and elevates hippocampal acetylcholine in young rats. Pharmacol Biochem Behav 1991;39(3):781–6.

73. Mason RP, Leeds PR, Jacob RF, et al. Inhibition of excessive neuronal apoptosis by the calcium antagonist amlodipine and antioxidants in cerebellar granule cells. J Neurochem 1999;72(4):1448–56.

74. Morich FJ, Bieber F, Lewis JM, et al. Nimodipine in the treatment of probable alzheimer's disease. Clin Drug Invest 1996;11(4):185–95.

75. Sandin M, Jasmin S, Levere TE. Aging and cognition: facilitation of recent memory in aged nonhuman primates by nimodipine. Neurobiol Aging 1990;11(5):573–5.

76. Kawahara M, Kuroda Y. Intracellular calcium changes in neuronal cells induced by alzheimer's ß-amyloid protein are blocked by estradiol and cholesterol. Cell Mol Neurobiol 2001;21(1):1–13.

77. Iadecola C, Park L, Capone C. Threats to the mind. Stroke 2009;40(3_suppl_1):S40–4.

78. Cao LL, Guan PP, Liang YY, et al. Calcium ions stimulate the hyperphosphorylation of tau by activating microsomal prostaglandin e synthase 1. Front Aging Neurosci 2019;11. Available at: https://www.frontiersin.org/articles/10.3389/fnagi.2019.00108. [Accessed 29 February 2024].

79. Rashid T, Li K, Toledo JB, et al. Association of intensive vs standard blood pressure control with regional changes in cerebral small vessel disease biomarkers: post hoc secondary analysis of the SPRINT MIND randomized clinical trial. JAMA Netw Open 2023;6(3):e231055.

80. Nasrallah IM, Pajewski NM, Auchus AP, et al. Association of intensive vs standard blood pressure control with cerebral white matter lesions. JAMA 2019;322(6): 524–34.

81. de Havenon A, Majersik JJ, Tirschwell DL, et al. Blood pressure, glycemic control, and white matter hyperintensity progression in type 2 diabetics. Neurology 2019; 92(11):e1168–75.

82. Zhao B, Jia W, Yuan Y, et al. Effects of intensive blood pressure control on cognitive function in patients with cerebral small vessel disease. J Stroke Cerebrovasc Dis 2023;32(9). https://doi.org/10.1016/j.jstrokecerebrovasdis.2023.107289.

83. White WB, Wakefield DB, Moscufo N, et al. Effects of intensive versus standard ambulatory blood pressure control on cerebrovascular outcomes in older people (INFINITY). Circulation 2019;140(20):1626–35.

84. Alpérovitch A, Blachier M, Soumaré A, et al. Blood pressure variability and risk of dementia in an elderly cohort, the three-city study. Alzheimers Dement 2014;10(5 Suppl):S330–7.

85. Yano Y, Ning H, Allen N, et al. Long-term blood pressure variability throughout young adulthood and cognitive function in midlife. Hypertension 2014;64(5): 983–8.

86. Yano Y, Griswold M, Wang W, et al. Long-term blood pressure level and variability from midlife to later life and subsequent cognitive change: the aric neurocognitive study. J Am Heart Assoc 2018;7(15):e009578.

87. de Havenon A, Anadani M, Prabhakaran S, et al. Increased blood pressure variability and the risk of probable dementia or mild cognitive impairment: a post hoc analysis of the sprint mind trial. J Am Heart Assoc 2021;10(18):e022206.

88. de Heus RAA, Tzourio C, Lee EJL, et al. Association between blood pressure variability with dementia and cognitive impairment: a systematic review and meta-analysis. Hypertension 2021;78(5):1478–89.

89. Waldstein SR, Rice SC, Thayer JF, et al. Pulse pressure and pulse wave velocity are related to cognitive decline in the baltimore longitudinal study of aging. Hypertension 2008;51(1):99–104.

90. Laurent S, Cockcroft J, Van Bortel L, et al. Expert consensus document on arterial stiffness: methodological issues and clinical applications. Eur Heart J 2006; 27(21):2588–605.

91. Tuday E, Heredia CP, Moreno D, et al. The role of vascular aging in the development of hypertension. Clin Geriatr Med 2024;40(4).

92. McDade E, Sun Z, Lee CW, et al. The association between pulse pressure change and cognition in late life: age and where you start matters. Alzheimer's Dementia: Diagnosis, Assessment & Disease Monitoring 2016;4:56–66.

93. Nagai M, Hoshide S, Ishikawa J, et al. Ambulatory blood pressure as an independent determinant of brain atrophy and cognitive function in elderly hypertension. J Hypertens 2008;26(8):1636–41.

94. Whelton PK, Carey RM, Aronow WS, et al. 2017 ACC/AHA/AAPA/ABC/ACPM/AGS/APhA/ASH/ASPC/NMA/PCNA guideline for the prevention, detection, evaluation, and management of high blood pressure in adults. J Am Coll Cardiol 2018; 71(19):e127–248.

95. SPRINT Research Group, Wright JT, Williamson JD, Ambrosius WT, et al. A randomized trial of intensive versus standard blood-pressure control. N Engl J Med 2015;373(22):2103–16.

96. Williamson JD, Miller ME, Bryan RN, et al. The action to control cardiovascular risk in diabetes memory in diabetes study (ACCORD-MIND): rationale, design, and methods. Am J Cardiol 2007;99(12A):112i–22i.

97. Lyon M, Fullerton JL, Kennedy S, et al. Hypertension & dementia: pathophysiology & potential utility of antihypertensives in reducing disease burden. Pharmacol Therapeut 2024;253:108575.

98. Daugherty AM. Hypertension-related risk for dementia: a summary review with future directions. Semin Cell Dev Biol 2021;116:82–9.

Nonpharmacologic Management of Hypertension in Older Adults

Carter Baughman, MD[a], Yusi Gong, MD[a], Yingfei Wu, MD, MPH[b],
Emma Hanlon, MD[a], Stephen Juraschek, MD, PhD[a],*

KEYWORDS

- Hypertension • Older adults • Nonpharmacologic management
- Lifestyle interventions • Blood pressure management

KEY POINTS

- Hypertension is prevalent among older adults and contributes to major adverse cardiovascular events.
- Nonpharmacologic interventions such as reduced sodium intake, a healthy diet, physical activity, and weight loss among those with obesity are effective in lowering blood pressure among older adults and should be emphasized in this population.
- Nonpharmacologic interventions can complement antihypertensive medications to decrease the risk of cardiovascular events.

INTRODUCTION

Hypertension affects 75% of adults over 60 years in the United States and is one of the strongest risk factors for major adverse cardiovascular events such as myocardial infarction, stroke, and heart failure.[1–3] Untreated, chronic elevations in blood pressure (BP) are a major risk factor for cardiovascular disease-related hospitalizations and death, cognitive decline, loss of autonomy, and overall lower health-related quality of life in older age.[2,4,5]

Nonpharmacologic lifestyle interventions represent important preventive and adjunct strategies in the treatment of hypertension. They are particularly relevant for older adults due to their pleiotropic benefits beyond cardiovascular disease and ability to be complementary with pharmacologic treatments. Owing to higher prevalence of comorbid conditions and concomitant frailty, nonpharmacologic interventions should be emphasized to decrease polypharmacy and its risks.[6] While

[a] Department of Medicine, Beth Israel Deaconess Medical Center, Harvard Medical School, Deaconess Building, Suite 306, One Deaconess Road, Boston, MA 02215, USA; [b] Department of Medicine, Massachusetts General Hospital, Harvard Medical School, Boston, MA, USA
* Corresponding author. 330 Brookline Avenue, CO-1309, #217, Boston, MA 02215.
E-mail address: sjurasch@bidmc.harvard.edu

Clin Geriatr Med 40 (2024) 615–628
https://doi.org/10.1016/j.cger.2024.04.013
0749-0690/24/© 2024 Elsevier Inc. All rights reserved.
geriatric.theclinics.com

there are an increasing number of pharmacologic options to treat traditional lifestyle contributors to hypertension (eg, obesity), here, we examine nonpharmacologic interventions with the strongest evidence for hypertension management (**Table 1**).

NUTRITION
Sodium Intake and Salt Sensitivity

The American Heart Association (AHA) recommends less than 2300 mg of sodium intake per day for adults and less than 1500 mg for people with hypertension.[7–9] Older adults, on average, consume less sodium than younger adults, but still far surpass recommendations; 94% of men and 78% of women greater than 60 years exceed 2300 mg per day.[9] When estimating sodium density consumption, which accounts for kilocalorie intake and is more strongly associated with BP, estimates are worse. A national study found that only 5.1% of adults consume less than 1.1 mg/kcal of sodium per day (ie, 2300 mg of sodium in a 2100 kcal diet), and these rates are similar in adults 60 to 80 years.[10]

The majority of sodium consumption in the United States is a result of processed foods, and adults aged ≥60 years have the highest rates of ultra-processed food consumption (57% per kcal).[11,12] Older adults, particularly frail individuals and those in

Table 1	
Nonpharmacologic interventions for decreasing blood pressure among older adults	
Intervention	**Summary of Recommendations**
Sodium Reduction	<1500 mg/day, or at least 1000 mg/day reduction in the general adult population, extrapolated to older adults (AHA) <1800 mg/day in older adults (TONE trial)
Dietary Patterns	Eating a diet rich in fruits, vegetables, and low-fat dairy, and low in total fat, saturated fat and cholesterol (DASH trial) Mediterranean diet (PREDIMED trial) Potassium-rich diet (SSaSS trial)
Alcohol	≤2 drinks/day in men, ≤1 drink/day in women (AHA)
Physical Activity	150 min per week of MVPA, defined as >3 metabolic equivalents of task (CDC) High-intensity interval training Moderate-intensity activity (eg, walking) Resistance training (eg, weight lifting) Decreasing sedentary time if MVPA is unachievable
Obesity	Targeted weight loss for those with obesity, along with adequate physical activity and nutrition intake (TONE trial)
Sleep	CPAP use is likely beneficial those with sleep apnea and resistant hypertension
Stress	More studies are needed to identify the role of stress reduction techniques on hypertension in the aging population; however, multidisciplinary management seems beneficial
Social Considerations	Address unique challenges faced by older patients when managing hypertension, from social determinants of health to social and financial support

Abbreviations: AHA, American Heart Association; CDC, Centers for Disease Control and Prevention; CPAP, continuous positive airway pressure; DASH, dietary approach to stopping hypertension; MVPA, moderate-to-vigorous physical activity; PREDIMED, Prevention with Mediterranean Diet; SSaSS, salt substitute and stroke study; TONE, trial of nonpharmacologic intervention in the elderly.

assisted living, often rely on others for food preparation and "ready meals."[13] This limits food choices and increases exposure to sodium-dense, processed foods. Food insecurity has increased among adults greater than 60 years from 5.5% to 12.4% between 2007 and 2016,[14] further exacerbating the reduced choice and low-quality diets common among older adults.

Aging is also associated with a decline in orosensory functions. Impaired taste is present in 0.93% of the general population but increases to 5.1% among adults aged 60 to 69 years and up to 22% of elderly nursing home residents.[15] The perception of bland taste leading to increased savory food is hypothesized, though evidence is mixed on the degree to which this impacts food choice.[15]

Salt sensitivity is a major contributor of hypertension among older adults. One study compared salt sensitivity, defined as a decrease in BP by greater than 10 mm Hg after sodium and volume depletion, in normotensive and hypertensive adults over and under 40 years of age.[16] They found significantly higher salt sensitivity among older adults. The mechanism of salt sensitivity is complex but is thought to occur in part due to reduced ability to excrete a salt load from declining renal function as well as endothelial dysfunction.[17]

Sodium Reduction

For reasons discussed earlier, sodium reduction represents an important, evidence-based strategy for nonpharmacologic management of hypertension in older adults (**Fig. 1**). The landmark Dietary Approach to Stop Hypertension (DASH)-Sodium trial showed the efficacy of a reduced sodium diet on hypertension. Participants (mean [SD] age of 47 [10] years) randomized to a reduced sodium DASH diet had significantly lower BP versus control, and the effect was more pronounced in participants with hypertension.[18]

A large meta-analysis reviewing dietary sodium and BP further supports a linear relationship between sodium intake and reduction in both systolic BP (SBP) and diastolic BP (DBP), with a more pronounced effects among participants with a higher baseline BP.[19]

The Trial of Nonpharmacologic Intervention in the Elderly (TONE) evaluated sodium reduction on BP specifically among community dwelling adults aged 60 to 80 years who were actively treated for hypertension.[20] They found that sodium reduction significantly decreased BP and reduced antihypertensive medication utilization.

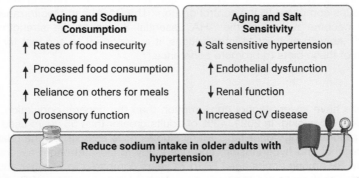

Fig. 1. Relationship between sodium intake, salt sensitivity, and importance of reducing sodium consumption among older adults with hypertension. CV, cardiovascular. (Created with Biorender.com.)

Smaller trials have been conducted in senior living facilities and shown similar trends in sodium reduction. One study randomized 20 adults ≥60 years to meal plans with different sodium densities (<0.95 mg/kcal vs >2 mg/kcal) and found lower SBP among the low sodium group, though it was not statistically significant. Overall, the study showed that implementing a low-sodium meal plan in a senior living facility has a strong suggestion toward lowering SBP in this population with minimal side effects.[21]

Dietary Approach to Stopping Hypertension

The DASH trial showed that a dietary pattern high in fruits, vegetables, and low-fat dairy and low in total fat, saturated fat, and cholesterol led to significant reductions in BP.[22] In this trial, participants with chronic hypertension received a diet rich in fruits and vegetables, a combination (DASH) diet, or a control diet; the trial found a more significant reduction in SBP and DBP from the DASH versus control diet. The DASH diet was higher in potassium, calcium, and magnesium than the control diet, which may be important contributors to the observed decrease in BP.

Potassium

Potassium-rich diets are associated with lower BP. Many mechanisms have been proposed, including increased sodium excretion and decreasing salt sensitivity which could be particularly impactful for older adults.[23] The Salt Substitute and Stroke Study (SSaSS) evaluated the impact of a potassium–sodium salt substitute (75% NaCl, 25% KCl) among hypertensive adults ≥60 years and found significantly lower BP, stroke, and other adverse cardiovascular events among the salt substituted group.[24] Individualized recommendations should be made for patients at risk for hyperkalemia (ie, advanced kidney disease, potassium-sparing diuretics), but in general, there is strong evidence that both a lower sodium and higher potassium intake may be beneficial for lowering BP among older adults.

Prevention with Mediterranean Diet

The Prevention with Mediterranean Diet (PREDIMED) trial evaluated adults aged 55 to 80 years with cardiovascular risk factors randomized to a Mediterranean diet with extra virgin olive oil, a Mediterranean diet with mixed nuts, or low-fat control diet. They found that all 3 interventions lowered BP with the 2 Mediterranean groups significantly decreasing DBP compared to the control diet.[25] Further analysis from this trial showed that participants had lower risk of overall major cardiovascular events in the Mediterranean groups compared to the control group.[26] The DASH and Mediterranean style diet have become a part of the AHA Essential 8 due to the strength of this evidence.[27] As with all lifestyle interventions, it is important to account for cultural adaptation of these diets to promote adherence.[28]

ALCOHOL

Older adults have lower alcohol consumption than the general population, though prevalence is increasing. In 2021, 42% of adults greater than 65 years used alcohol and 11% reported binge drinking.[29] Many studies have established the relationship between alcohol and hypertension, and one study found a stronger association of alcohol and BP among adults aged 50 to 74 years compared to younger adults.[30,31] A large meta-analysis found that reducing alcohol led to significant BP reductions among those who drank greater than 2 drinks per day and was strongest among those who had 6 or more drinks per day and cut their intake in half.[32] The AHA guidelines for alcohol intake among older adults mirror the general population, recommending 2 or less drinks in men and ≤1 drink in women per day.[8]

PHYSICAL ACTIVITY

Participation in physical activity (PA) has been shown to increase muscle function and balance, decrease pain, counteract frailty-related physical and cognitive impairment, and reduce BP.[33,34] Regular PA is a cornerstone for both the prevention and treatment of hypertension.[34] BP has been shown to decrease for up to 22 hours after exercise, a phenomenon thought to be due to sympathetic nerve inactivity, reduced vascular tone, and vasodilation.[35] In the long term, regular exercise improves cardiac function and metabolism.[36]

For older adults, the Centers for Disease Control and Prevention recommends at least 150 minutes of moderate-to-vigorous PA (MVPA) weekly (>3 metabolic equivalents of task [METs]) with at least 2 days per week of muscle strengthening activities. Any activity is better than none, and there is a graded benefit in health outcomes with increased activity.[37] Despite the known benefits of exercise on mortality, joint pain, and overall well-being, only 10% to 15% of adults greater than 65 years achieve these recommendations.[37,38] Decreased PA uptake is likely contributed by reduced physical fitness, functional limitations, and chronic disease or pain associated with advanced age.[38,39] Other barriers include fear of falling, depressive symptoms, lack of time, and general disinterest in activity.[39]

Older adults are a varied group with a range of chronic diseases and frailty states, and finding effective interventions to address these barriers is crucial. Multiple exercise modalities, for example, water-based exercise,[40] have been shown to reduce BP among older adults. High-intensity interval training is a time-efficient, safe modality of exercise characterized by bursts of vigorous activity followed by periods of rest or low-intensity activity, while moderate-intensity activity such as walking is an aerobic activity at sustained intensity.[41] Both are effective in BP reduction, especially among older adults with a higher baseline BP.[42–45] Resistance training is also important in preventing osteopenia, maintaining strength, and improving balance, and has been shown to have favorable BP effects among older adults.[46]

Sedentary time, defined as waking behavior with energy expenditure less than 1.5 METs, is associated with progression of chronic disease, frailty, and all-cause mortality among older adults.[37] Decreasing sedentary time improves cardiovascular disease risk factors independent of PA and may decrease BP.[47] Reducing sedentary time may be more feasible for some older adults than increasing PA and remains an important nonpharmacologic antihypertensive treatment.

OBESITY

Obesity is a risk factor for hypertension among older adults via impaired vascular function, activation of the sympathetic nervous system and the renin–angiotensin–aldosterone system, as well as other inflammatory pathways.[48] Adipose tissue is also associated with increased arterial stiffness, and weight loss has been shown to reverse endothelial dysfunction.[49,50] Therefore, targeting obesity through both pharmacologic and nonpharmacologic interventions have been shown to improve BP among hypertensive patients.

Intentional weight loss is generally recommended for older obese individuals with hypertension, especially for those with secondary hypertension attributed to obesity, although specific weight loss targets vary.[3,8] Studies of weight loss effects on BP are more limited in older populations than the general population but still demonstrate an association with BP reduction.[51] In the TONE trial, weight loss reduced BP among older adults and reduced hypertension treatment.[20]

One major nonpharmacologic, surgical treatment shown to improve hypertension control among older obese patients is bariatric surgery. One meta-analysis of bariatric surgery in older adults revealed 42.5% resolution of hypertension.[52] However, geriatric bariatric surgery was also associated with higher rates of mortality and overall complications.[53] Considering the large potential benefit of bariatric surgery on hypertension and other health outcomes among obese older patients, careful risk and benefit assessments for this surgery along with other noninvasive methods of intentional weight loss should be discussed for individuals with comorbid hypertension, obesity, and related metabolic disorders.

It is important to note that excess weight loss among older adults has also been associated with harms, wherein higher body mass index has, at times, been shown to be protective against cardiovascular diseases including hypertension.[54] However, the evidence is conflicting and may be secondary to confounds such as sarcopenia, frailty, and unintentional weight loss.[55] Several studies have identified relationships between geriatric sarcopenia and sarcopenic obesity to hypertension and all-cause mortality.[56,57] Thus, utilizing more holistic measures of body composition such as waist circumference to measure visceral obesity, and concurrently encouraging PA and adequate nutritional intake to maintain muscle mass and prevent frailty, may reflect more appropriate strategies when counseling intentional weight loss to improve hypertension for older adults with obesity.

SLEEP

The relationship between sleep and hypertension among aging adults is complex, making targeted interventions challenging. Interventions have focused on sleep type, duration, and conditions affecting sleep. However, many relationships between sleep and hypertension in the general population are not directly applicable to older adults.

Sleep is divided into rapid eye movement (REM) and non-REM sleep. Within non-REM sleep, slow wave sleep is associated with elevated vagal tone and reduced sympathetic activity, and in one study of men ≥65 years, decreased slow wave sleep was associated with a higher risk of incident hypertension.[58] In contrast, shorter sleep duration is not associated with greater risk of incident or prevalent hypertension among adults greater than 65 years despite this observation among younger adults.[59] Several reasons for the differences in importance of sleep duration with respect to hypertension among older adults include shorter lifespans for those with multimorbidity and lower survival, sleep pattern changes with aging, and increased opportunities for daytime napping among older adults.[60] Thus, while increased restorative sleep may have benefits for improving risk of hypertension, this does not extrapolate to overall sleep duration.

Etiology of disrupted sleep is also important for older adults with respect to hypertension. In obstructive sleep apnea (OSA), or sleep-disordered breathing, it is hypothesized that intermittent episodes of hypoxia have effects on chemoreceptors and alterations in autonomic activity which increases risk of hypertension.[61] However, evidence is inconsistent. While some studies have found no association between sleep-disordered breathing and hypertension among older adults (≥60 years), others report an association between nocturnal nondipping and sleep-disordered breathing among older adults.[62,63] Moreover, it is unclear whether treatment with continuous positive airway pressure (CPAP) consistently reduces BP. One meta-analysis found that

CPAP therapy improved 24 hour BP in those with OSA and resistant hypertension, and that older age was associated with greater improvement in DBP.[64] However, another analysis found that in adults ≥80 years, CPAP use did not improve BP control.[65]

It should be noted that hypertension itself may contribute to fragmented sleep. Nocturnal hypertension or nondipping has been associated with nocturnal polyuria, which is a common cause of nighttime awakening.[66,67] Moreover, hypertension treatment overnight or with CPAP can reduce nocturia.[68] This could account for the impression that sleep may be causing hypertension, when the reverse may be true in some cases. For these patients, controlling hypertension may be necessary to improve sleep (rather than improving sleep for hypertension), but more work is needed to confirm this hypothesis.

STRESS

In the general population, cardiovascular disease is associated with psychosocial factors including acute and chronic stress, depression, anxiety, and isolation.[69–71] Stress is thought to stimulate the sympathetic nervous system, increasing heart rate, BP, and endothelial dysfunction and injury.[69]

There are examples in the literature whereby both acute stress events (eg, earthquake) and chronic stress (eg, being a spousal caregiver) were identified as risk factors for hypertension among older adults.[72,73] However, interventions to reduce stress have had inconsistent effects on BP among older adults. One primary care-based intervention for multidisciplinary management of hypertension in older adults showed promising benefits with both reduced perceived stress and improved SBP.[74] Moreover, a meta-analysis evaluated the effect of stress reduction interventions including biofeedback, progressive muscle relaxation, or a combination of different techniques, suggesting that stress reduction techniques lowered BP in those with hypertension, though not specific to older adults.[75] Moreover, yoga and tai chi have also seemed to lower BP, although there are substantial methodological differences across trials.[76,77] Nevertheless, the Trials of Hypertension Prevention trial found no benefit from stress reduction on BP, attesting to the extensive heterogeneity of both interventions and individual responses.[78] Overall, while acute and chronic stress likely have an adversarial effect on BP, further research on targeted interventions for the aging population is needed.

SOCIAL CONSIDERATIONS

Older adults face unique social factors affecting their ability to manage chronic diseases such as hypertension, including social isolation, financial hardship, and lack of independence.[79] Social determinants of health, including food insecurity, unstable housing, and financial stress also affect health behaviors among older adults.[80] Given the increased prevalence of social isolation and dependency faced by older adults, one important association linked to improved hypertension control in this population is social support. Social isolation among older adults has been associated with behaviors that increase health risk and higher inflammatory markers,[81] while social participation has been associated with decreased risk of hypertension.[82] Specifically, observational studies have shown that family and community support is associated with the promotion of health behaviors as well as lower BP among older adults, especially for those from minoritized backgrounds.[83,84]

In addition to identifying social factors, older subpopulations also warrant special considerations. There remain racial and ethnic health inequities in geriatric hypertension, including increased prevalence and poorer management of hypertension, which

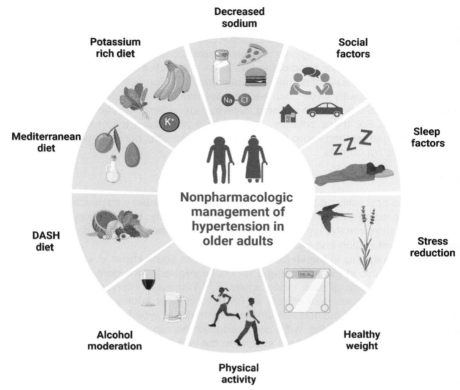

Fig. 2. Nonpharmacologic management strategies to treat hypertension in older adults. (Created with Biorender.com.)

remain apparent even after adjustment for socioeconomic status and other comorbidities.[85,86] Generic hypertension interventions have, at times, been less efficacious among minoritized groups.[86,87] Conversely, culturally tailored behavioral interventions for ethnic subgroups improve efficacy.[88,89]

There are many other older population groups that may require individualized attention in managing hypertension, beyond the scope of this review, including those with comorbid mental health and cognitive disorders, those living in assisted living facilities, and those with language preferences other than English. Given the multitude of social barriers faced by older adults when managing hypertension, it is imperative for clinicians to recognize and address these barriers to facilitate hypertension control.

SUMMARY

Nonpharmacologic management of hypertension among older adults includes a range of evidence-based tools. In this review, the authors discuss multiple lifestyle and social interventions to enhance hypertension management among this population (**Fig. 2**). Nonpharmacologic interventions are most useful in combination and with or without pharmacologic therapies.[90,91] When utilized in the context of individual patients' social backgrounds, these interventions can significantly lower BP and improve cardiovascular outcomes in the geriatric population.

CLINICS CARE POINTS

- Decreasing sodium, increasing potassium, and the DASH and Mediterranean diets have strong evidence to reduce BP among older adults.
- Aerobic and resistance training in sedentary hypertensive older adults is effective in lowering BP, improving physical function, and preventing falls.
- Targeting weight loss for those with obesity, in conjunction with PA and healthy nutrition, has a strong association with decreased BP among older adults with hypertension.
- Improving sleep quality, reducing chronic stress, and addressing social factors affecting older adults are additional ways to target BP reduction among older adults.

DISCLOSURE

The work of S. Juraschek is supported by R01MD016068, R01HL153191, and R01HL158622. The work of Y. Wu is supported by HRSA, United States grant number 5T32HP42013.

REFERENCES

1. Ostchega Y, Fryar CD, Nwankwo T, et al. Hypertension prevalence among adults aged 18 and over: United States, 2017-2018. NCHS Data Brief 2020;(364):1–8.
2. Fuchs FD, Whelton PK. High blood pressure and cardiovascular disease. Hypertens Dallas Tex 1979. 2020;75(2):285–92.
3. Benetos A, Petrovic M, Strandberg T. Hypertension management in older and frail older patients. Circ Res 2019;124(7):1045–60.
4. Vu THT, Zhao L, Liu L, et al. Favorable cardiovascular health at young and middle ages and dementia in older age-the CHA study. J Am Heart Assoc 2019;8(1): e009730.
5. Daviglus ML, Liu K, Pirzada A, et al. Favorable cardiovascular risk profile in middle age and health-related quality of life in older age. Arch Intern Med 2003; 163(20):2460–8.
6. Fried TR, O'Leary J, Towle V, et al. Health outcomes associated with polypharmacy in community-dwelling older adults: a systematic review. J Am Geriatr Soc 2014;62(12):2261–72.
7. Lloyd-Jones DM, Hong Y, Labarthe D, et al. Defining and setting national goals for cardiovascular health promotion and disease reduction. Circulation 2010; 121(4):586–613.
8. 2017 ACC/AHA/AAPA/ABC/ACPM/AGS/APhA/ASH/ASPC/NMA/PCNA guideline for the prevention, detection, evaluation, and management of high blood pressure in adults: a report of the american college of cardiology/american heart association task force on clinical practice guidelines. Hypertension 2018. https://doi.org/10.1161/HYP.0000000000000065.
9. U.S. Department of Agriculture and U.S. Department of Health and Human Services. Dietary Guidelines for Americans, 2020-2025. 9th Edition. 2020. Available at: DietaryGuidelines.gov.
10. Hu JR, Sahni S, Mukamal KJ, et al. Dietary sodium intake and sodium density in the United States: estimates from NHANES 2005–2006 and 2015–2016. Am J Hypertens 2020;33(9):825–30.
11. Harnack LJ, Cogswell ME, Shikany JM, et al. Sources of sodium in US adults from 3 geographic regions. Circulation 2017;135(19):1775–83.

12. Juul F, Parekh N, Martinez-Steele E, et al. Ultra-processed food consumption among US adults from 2001 to 2018. Am J Clin Nutr 2022;115(1):211–21.
13. Hoffman R. Micronutrient deficiencies in the elderly – could ready meals be part of the solution? J Nutr Sci 2017;6:e2.
14. Leung CW, Wolfson JA. Food insecurity among older adults: ten-year national trends and associations with diet quality. J Am Geriatr Soc 2021;69(4):964–71.
15. Song X, Giacalone D, Bølling Johansen SM, et al. Changes in orosensory perception related to aging and strategies for counteracting its influence on food preferences among older adults. Trends Food Sci Technol 2016;53:49–59.
16. Luft FC, Weinberger MH, Fineberg NS, et al. Effects of age on renal sodium homeostasis and its relevance to sodium sensitivity. Am J Med 1987;82(1B):9–15.
17. Choi HY, Park HC, Ha SK. Salt sensitivity and hypertension: a paradigm shift from kidney malfunction to vascular endothelial dysfunction. Electrolytes Blood Press E BP 2015;13(1):7–16.
18. Sacks FM, Svetkey LP, Vollmer WM, et al. Effects on blood pressure of reduced dietary sodium and the dietary approaches to stop hypertension (DASH) diet. N Engl J Med 2001;344(1):3–10.
19. Filippini T, Malavolti M, Whelton P, et al. Blood pressure effects of sodium reduction: dose–response meta-analysis of experimental studies. Circulation 2021;143: 1542–67.
20. Whelton PK, Appel LJ, Espeland MA, et al. Sodium reduction and weight loss in the treatment of hypertension in older personsa randomized controlled trial of nonpharmacologic interventions in the elderly (TONE). JAMA 1998;279(11):839–46.
21. Juraschek SP, Millar CL, Foley A, et al. The effects of a low sodium meal plan on blood pressure in older adults: the sotrue randomized feasibility trial. Nutrients 2021;13(3):964.
22. Appel LJ, Moore TJ, Obarzanek E, et al. A clinical trial of the effects of dietary patterns on blood pressure. N Engl J Med 1997;336(16):1117–24.
23. Ellison DH, Welling P. Insights into salt handling and blood pressure. N Engl J Med 2021;385(21):1981–93.
24. Neal B, Wu Y, Feng X, et al. Effect of salt substitution on cardiovascular events and death. N Engl J Med 2021;385(12):1067–77.
25. Toledo E, Hu FB, Estruch R, et al. Effect of the mediterranean diet on blood pressure in the PREDIMED trial: results from a randomized controlled trial. BMC Med 2013;11(1):207.
26. Estruch R, Ros E, Salas-Salvadó J, et al. Primary prevention of cardiovascular disease with a mediterranean diet supplemented with extra-virgin olive oil or nuts. N Engl J Med 2018;378(25):e34.
27. Lloyd-Jones DM, Allen NB, Anderson CAM, et al. Life's essential 8: updating and enhancing the American Heart Association's construct of cardiovascular health: a presidential advisory from the American Heart Association. Circulation 2022; 146(5):e18–43.
28. Woodside J, Young IS, McKinley MC. Culturally adapting the Mediterranean Diet pattern – a way of promoting more 'sustainable' dietary change? Br J Nutr 2022; 128(4):693–703.
29. Results from the 2021 National Survey on Drug Use and Health: Detailed Tables.
30. Fuchs FD, Chambless LE, Whelton PK, et al. Alcohol consumption and the incidence of hypertension. Hypertension 2001;37(5):1242–50.
31. Fortmann SP, Haskell WL, Vranizan K, et al. The association of blood pressure and dietary alcohol: differences by age, sex, and estrogen use1. Am J Epidemiol 1983;118(4):497–507.

32. Roerecke M, Kaczorowski J, Tobe SW, et al. The effect of a reduction in alcohol consumption on blood pressure: a systematic review and meta-analysis. Lancet Public Health 2017;2(2):e108–20.

33. Angulo J, El Assar M, Álvarez-Bustos A, et al. Physical activity and exercise: strategies to manage frailty. Redox Biol 2020;35:101513.

34. Saco-Ledo G, Valenzuela PL, Ruiz-Hurtado G, et al. Exercise reduces ambulatory blood pressure in patients with hypertension: a systematic review and meta-analysis of randomized controlled trials. J Am Heart Assoc 2020;9(24):e018487.

35. Brandão RMUP, Alves MJNN, Braga AMFW, et al. Postexercise blood pressure reduction in elderly hypertensive patients. J Am Coll Cardiol 2002;39(4):676–82.

36. Fiuza-Luces C, Santos-Lozano A, Joyner M, et al. Exercise benefits in cardiovascular disease: beyond attenuation of traditional risk factors. Nat Rev Cardiol 2018;15(12):731–43.

37. CDC. Physical activity guidelines for Americans 2nd edition. 2018. Available at: https://health.gov/sites/default/files/2019-09/Physical_Activity_Guidelines_2nd_edition.pdf.

38. Elgaddal N, Kramarow EA, Reuben C. Physical activity among adults aged 18 and over: United States, 2020. Hyattsville, MD: Centers of Disease Control and Prevention; 2022. https://doi.org/10.15620/cdc:120213.

39. Macera CA, Cavanaugh A, Bellettiere J. State of the art review: physical activity and older adults. Am J Lifestyle Med 2017;11(1):42–57.

40. Ngomane AY, Fernandes B, Guimarães GV, et al. Hypotensive effect of heated water-based exercise in older individuals with hypertension. Int J Sports Med 2019;40(4):283–91.

41. Wewege MA, Ahn D, Yu J, et al. High-intensity interval training for patients with cardiovascular disease-is it safe? a systematic review. J Am Heart Assoc 2018; 7(21):e009305.

42. Pinto A, Di Raimondo D, Tuttolomondo A, et al. Twenty-four hour ambulatory blood pressure monitoring to evaluate effects on blood pressure of physical activity in hypertensive patients. Clin J Sport Med 2006;16(3):238–43.

43. Kerr J, Rosenberg D, Millstein RA, et al. Cluster randomized controlled trial of a multilevel physical activity intervention for older adults. Int J Behav Nutr Phys Act 2018;15(1):32.

44. He LI, Wei WR, Can Z. Effects of 12-week brisk walking training on exercise blood pressure in elderly patients with essential hypertension: a pilot study. Clin Exp Hypertens N Y N 1993. 2018;40(7):673–9.

45. Carpes L, Costa R, Schaarschmidt B, et al. High-intensity interval training reduces blood pressure in older adults: a systematic review and meta-analysis. Exp Gerontol 2022;158:111657.

46. Henkin JS, Pinto RS, Machado CLF, et al. Chronic effect of resistance training on blood pressure in older adults with prehypertension and hypertension: a systematic review and meta-analysis. Exp Gerontol 2023;177:112193.

47. Lee PH, Wong FKY. The association between time spent in sedentary behaviors and blood pressure: a systematic review and meta-analysis. Sports Med Auckl NZ 2015;45(6):867–80.

48. Kotchen TA. Obesity-related hypertension: epidemiology, pathophysiology, and clinical management. Am J Hypertens 2010;23(11):1170–8.

49. Csipo T, Fulop GA, Lipecz A, et al. Short-term weight loss reverses obesity-induced microvascular endothelial dysfunction. GeroScience 2018;40(3):337–46.

50. Rider OJ, Tayal U, Francis JM, et al. The effect of obesity and weight loss on aortic pulse wave velocity as assessed by magnetic resonance imaging. Obes Silver Spring Md 2010;18(12):2311–6.

51. Gill LE, Bartels SJ, Batsis JA. Weight management in older adults. Curr Obes Rep 2015;4(3):379–88.

52. Giordano S, Vvictorzon M. Bariatric surgery in elderly patients: a systematic review. Clin Interv Aging 2015;10:1627–35.

53. Giordano S, Victorzon M. Laparoscopic roux-en-y gastric bypass in elderly patients (60 years or older): a meta-analysis of comparative studies. Scand J Surg 2018;107(1):6–13.

54. Tutor AW, Lavie CJ, Kachur S, et al. Updates on obesity and the obesity paradox in cardiovascular diseases. Prog Cardiovasc Dis 2023;78:2–10.

55. Miller SL, Wolfe RR. The danger of weight loss in the elderly. J Nutr Health Aging 2008;12(7):487–91.

56. Qu Q, Guo Q, Sun J, et al. Low lean mass with obesity in older adults with hypertension: prevalence and association with mortality rate. BMC Geriatr 2023; 23(1):619.

57. Quan Y, Wang C, Wang L, et al. Geriatric sarcopenia is associated with hypertension: a systematic review and meta-analysis. J Clin Hypertens 2023;25(9): 808–16.

58. Fung MM, Peters K, Redline S, et al. Decreased slow wave sleep increases risk of developing hypertension in elderly men. Hypertension 2011;58(4):596–603.

59. Wang Q, Xi B, Liu M, et al. Short sleep duration is associated with hypertension risk among adults: a systematic review and meta-analysis. Hypertens Res 2012; 35(10):1012–8.

60. Gangwisch JE, Heymsfield SB, Boden-Albala B, et al. Short sleep duration as a risk factor for hypertension: analyses of the first national health and nutrition examination survey. Hypertension 2006;47(5):833–9.

61. Salman LA, Shulman R, Cohen JB. Obstructive sleep apnea, hypertension, and cardiovascular risk: epidemiology, pathophysiology, and management. Curr Cardiol Rep 2020;22(2):6.

62. Haas DC, Foster GL, Nieto FJ, et al. Age-dependent associations between sleep-disordered breathing and hypertension: importance of discriminating between systolic/diastolic hypertension and isolated systolic hypertension in the sleep heart health study. Circulation 2005;111(5):614–21.

63. Endeshaw YW, White WB, Kutner M, et al. Sleep-disordered breathing and 24-hour blood pressure pattern among older adults. J Gerontol A Biol Sci Med Sci 2009;64A(2):280–5.

64. Labarca G, Schmidt A, Dreyse J, et al. Efficacy of continuous positive airway pressure (CPAP) in patients with obstructive sleep apnea (OSA) and resistant hypertension (RH): systematic review and meta-analysis. Sleep Med Rev 2021;58: 101446.

65. Martinez-Garcia MA, Oscullo G, Ponce S, et al. Effect of continuous positive airway pressure in very elderly with moderate-to-severe obstructive sleep apnea pooled results from two multicenter randomized controlled trials. Sleep Med 2022;89:71–7.

66. Lombardo R, Tubaro A, Burkhard F. Nocturia: the complex role of the heart, kidneys, and bladder. Eur Urol Focus 2020;6(3):534–6.

67. Pesonen JS, Vernooij RWM, Cartwright R, et al. The impact of nocturia on falls and fractures: a systematic review and meta-analysis. J Urol 2020;203(4):674–83.

68. Juraschek SP, Cortez MM, Flack JM, et al. Orthostatic hypotension in adults with hypertension: a scientific statement from the american heart association. Hypertension 2024;81(3). https://doi.org/10.1161/HYP.0000000000000236.
69. Rozanski A, Blumenthal JA, Kaplan J. Impact of psychological factors on the pathogenesis of cardiovascular disease and implications for therapy. Circulation 1999;99(16):2192–217.
70. Figueredo VM. The time has come for physicians to take notice: the impact of psychosocial stressors on the heart. Am J Med 2009;122(8):704–12.
71. Dimsdale JE. Psychological stress and cardiovascular disease. J Am Coll Cardiol 2008;51(13):1237–46.
72. Kario K, Matsuo T, Kobayashi H, et al. Earthquake-induced potentiation of acute risk factors in hypertensive elderly patients: possible triggering of cardiovascular events after a major earthquake. J Am Coll Cardiol 1997;29(5):926–33.
73. Shaw WS, Patterson TL, Ziegler MG, et al. Accelerated risk of hypertensive blood pressure recordings among alzheimer caregivers. J Psychosom Res 1999;46(3):215–27.
74. Hajjar IM, Dickson B, Blackledge JL, et al. A multidisciplinary management program in primary care to improve hypertension control and healthy behaviors in elderly patients. J Am Geriatr Soc 2007;55(4):624–6.
75. Nagele E, Jeitler K, Horvath K, et al. Clinical effectiveness of stress-reduction techniques in patients with hypertension: systematic review and meta-analysis. J Hypertens 2014;32(10):1936–44.
76. Wang J, Xiong X, Liu W. Yoga for essential hypertension: a systematic review. In: Gonzalez GE, editor. PLoS ONE 2013;8(10):e76357.
77. Yeh GY, Wang C, Wayne PM, et al. The effect of tai chi exercise on blood pressure: a systematic review. Prev Cardiol 2008;11(2):82–9.
78. Batey D. Stress management intervention for primary prevention of hypertension detailed results from phase i of trials of hypertension prevention (TOHP-I). Ann Epidemiol 2000;10(1):45–58.
79. Miller KE, Zylstra RG, Standridge JB. The geriatric patient: a systematic approach to maintaining health. Am Fam Physician 2000;61(4):1089–104.
80. Sonnenblick R, Reilly A, Roye K, et al. Social determinants of health and hypertension control in adults with medicaid. J Prim Care Community Health 2022;13. 21501319221142426.
81. Shankar A, McMunn A, Banks J, et al. Loneliness, social isolation, and behavioral and biological health indicators in older adults. Health Psychol 2011;30(4):377–85.
82. Kamiya Y, Whelan B, Timonen V, et al. The differential impact of subjective and objective aspects of social engagement on cardiovascular risk factors. BMC Geriatr 2010;10(1):81.
83. Bell CN, Thorpe RJ, Laveist TA. Race/Ethnicity and hypertension: the role of social support. Am J Hypertens 2010;23(5):534–40.
84. Woods SB, Hiefner AR, Udezi V, et al. "They should walk with you": the perspectives of African Americans living with hypertension and their family members on disease self-management. Ethn Health 2023;28(3):373–98.
85. Gorman BK, Porter JR. Social networks and support, gender, and racial/ethnic disparities in hypertension among older adults. Popul Res Policy Rev 2011;30(6):885–911.
86. Delgado J, Jacobs EA, Lackland DT, et al. Differences in blood pressure control in a large population-based sample of older african americans and non-hispanic whites. J Gerontol Ser A 2012;67(11):1253–8.

87. Zullig LL, Liang Y, Vale Arismendez S, et al. Trajectory of systolic blood pressure in a low-income, racial-ethnic minority cohort with diabetes and baseline uncontrolled hypertension. J Clin Hypertens Greenwich Conn 2017;19(7):722–30.
88. Harrison TN, Zhou H, Wei R, et al. Blood pressure control among black and white adults following a quality improvement program in a large integrated health system. JAMA Netw Open 2023;6(1):e2249930.
89. Jackson GL, Oddone EZ, Olsen MK, et al. Racial differences in the effect of a telephone-delivered hypertension disease management program. J Gen Intern Med 2012;27(12):1682–9.
90. Appel LJ, Champagne CM, Harsha DW, et al. Effects of comprehensive lifestyle modification on blood pressure control: main results of the PREMIER clinical trial. JAMA 2003;289(16):2083–93.
91. Miller ER, Erlinger TP, Young DR, et al. Results of the diet, exercise, and weight loss intervention trial (DEW-IT). Hypertens Dallas Tex 1979 2002;40(5):612–8.

Pharmacologic Treatment of Hypertension in Older Adults

Oliver M. Todd, MBBS, PhD[a,b],*, Matthew Knight, MBBS[a],
Joshua A. Jacobs, PharmD[c], Catherine G. Derington, PharmD, MS[c],
James P. Sheppard, PhD[d], Adam P. Bress, PharmD, MS[c]

KEYWORDS

- Antihypertensive • Blood pressure • Frailty • Hypertension • Multimorbidity
- Aged pharmacotherapy

KEY POINTS

- Absolute cardiovascular benefits of lowering blood pressure with antihypertensives increase with age.
- Across the population, physiological changes with age affect the pharmacokinetic and pharmacodynamic properties of antihypertensive medications. As a result, while the risk of experiencing harm from antihypertensive medications is low, it also increases with age.
- Prediction models are available to identify older adults who are at high risk of adverse events to inform personalized treatment.
- Most clinical guidelines recommend the "start low, go slow" approach for initiating antihypertensive medication among older adults with consideration of frailty and multimorbidity guiding choice of the antihypertensive agent.

INTRODUCTION

In the United States, 3 out of 4 people will develop hypertension during their lifetime.[1] Hypertension is the leading modifiable risk factor for cardiovascular disease which

[a] Academic Unit for Ageing and Stroke Research, University of Leeds, Leeds, LS2 3AA, United Kingdom; [b] Bradford Institute for Health Research, Bradford Teaching Hospitals NHS Trust, Bradford BD9 6RJ, United Kingdom; [c] Intermountain Healthcare Department of Population Health Sciences, Spencer Fox Eccles School of Medicine, University of Utah, Salt Lake City, UT 84112, USA; [d] Nuffield Department of Primary Care Health Sciences, University of Oxford, Oxford OX2 6GG, United Kingdom
* Corresponding author. Room 5, Academic Unit for Ageing and Stroke Research, Bradford Institute for Health Research, Bradford Teaching Hospitals NHS Foundation Trust, Bradford BD96RJ.
E-mail address: o.todd@leeds.ac.uk
Twitter: @ToddOly (O.M.T.); @JoshJPharmD (J.A.J.)

Clin Geriatr Med 40 (2024) 629–644
https://doi.org/10.1016/j.cger.2024.04.004   **geriatric.theclinics.com**
0749-0690/24/© 2024 The Authors. Published by Elsevier Inc. This is an open access article under the CC BY license (http://creativecommons.org/licenses/by/4.0/).

accounts for approximately 30% of all deaths worldwide, and older adults represent those at the highest risk.[2–4] Nonpharmacological interventions are effective for lowering blood pressure (BP) yet difficult to achieve and maintain for most. Therefore, pharmacological therapy is usually needed to achieve BP control.

This article provides a review of the guidelines and the underlying evidence supporting recommendations for antihypertensive pharmacotherapy in older adults with hypertension. We review the most commonly used antihypertensive medication classes, relevant considerations for their use in older adults including the place for combination therapy, important adverse drug events (ADEs) to monitor and manage, and how to approach shared decision-making with older adults.

EVIDENCE SUPPORTING ANTIHYPERTENSIVE PHARMACOTHERAPY IN OLDER ADULTS

Increasing evidence supports the cardiovascular, renal, and neurovascular benefits of treating hypertension in older adults, emphasizing a thoughtful evaluation of risks and benefits.[5–7] Of note, all of the professional society guidelines since 2016 endorse the use of pharmacotherapy in older adult populations with hypertension.[8–14] However, guidelines vary widely on their age-based recommendations for thresholds for initiation and intensification of antihypertensive medication in older adults (**Fig. 1**).[15]

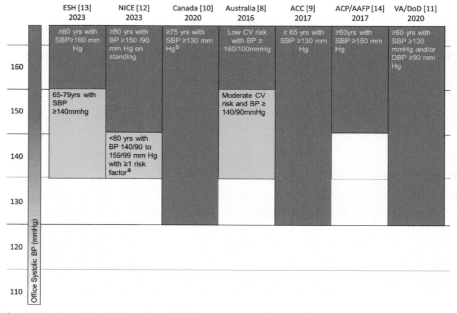

Fig. 1. Age-based variations in guideline recommendations for initiation of antihypertensive pharmacotherapy based on systolic blood pressure measurements among non-frail, non-institutionalized persons. [a]Additional risk factors include target organ damage, established atherosclerotic cardiovascular disease (ASCVD), renal disease, diabetes, estimated 10 year cardiovascular disease risk ≥10%. [b]High-risk conditions include age ≥75 years, clinical or subclinical ASCVD, chronic kidney disease, or 10 year Framingham risk score ≥15%. ACC, American College of Cardiology; ACP, American College of Physicians; AAFP, the American Academy of Family Physicians; ESH, European Society of Hypertension; NICE, the National Institute for Health and Care Excellence; VA/DoD, Veterans Affairs/Department of Defense.

The decision on which antihypertensive medication to prescribe to reduce cardio-vascular risk in older adults is generally perceived as less critical than achieving the target BP level. It is thought that the cardiovascular benefits result from the reduction in BP and less from direct effects of the medications independent of the BP change. There have been several randomized controlled trials (RCTs) of BP lowering with antihypertensive medication in older adults to inform treatment decisions **(Table 1)**.[5–7,16,17]

The Hypertension in the Very Elderly Trial (HYVET) and Systolic Blood Pressure Intervention Trial (SPRINT)-Senior are the two most widely cited RCTs to evaluate the effect of BP lowering in older adults. HYVET randomized patients age ≥80 years, with a sustained seated systolic BP (SBP) of 160 mm Hg or more, to receive either indapamide (with additional perindopril as required) or placebo.[5] Patients in the treatment arm had a 15 mm Hg lower reduction in SBP than the placebo group which resulted in a reduced rate of major adverse cardiovascular events (MACE), hazard ratio (HR) 0.66, 95% confidence interval (95% CI) 0.53 to 0.82, and a lower rate of serious ADEs ($P < .001$). SPRINT-Senior was a prespecified subgroup analysis of those age ≥75 years at baseline in SPRINT which randomized US adults age ≥50 years at high cardiovascular disease risk, without diabetes mellitus or stroke, to intensive (SBP target <120 mm Hg) versus standard (SBP <140 mm Hg) control.[6] In the age ≥75 years subgroup, participants in the intensive arm, compared to those in the standard treatment arm had a lower risk of MACE, HR 0.66, 95% CI 0.51 to 0.85 with no difference in the rate of serious ADEs HR 0.99, 95% CI 0.89 to 1.11.

In both HYVET and SPRINT-Senior, the investigators have examined the impact of frailty through retrospective analyses.[18,19] In both trials, the effect of the randomized intervention on MACE or ADEs was not different across frailty levels at baseline. Importantly, the subgroup living with more advanced frailty in both HYVET and SPRINT-Senior demonstrated a benefit of BP-lowering interventions on mortality and cardiovascular disease outcomes but did not have a higher risk of ADEs. However, there is some debate as to whether older adults living with severe frailty were represented in the trial population.[20]

In a meta-analysis incorporating individual patient-level data (IPD) from 358,707 participants across 51 RCTs, the benefits of BP lowering with antihypertensive medication were assessed in two distinct age cohorts: 54,016 participants aged 75 to 84 years and 4,788 participants aged ≥85 years.[21] The results demonstrated that each 5 mm Hg reduction in SBP consistently lowered the risk of MACE across all age groups, maintaining significance up to the age of 85 years. However, the magnitude of relative risk reduction varied by age, with the most substantial benefit observed in the youngest cohort and progressively smaller effects, accompanied by wider CIs, in older age groups. Specifically, the risks for MACE were as follows: HR 0.82, 95% CI 0.76 to 0.88 in adults less than 55 years; HR 0.91, 95% CI 0.88 to 0.95 for 55 to 64 years and similarly for 65 to 74 years; HR 0.91, 95% CI 0.87 to 0.96 for 75 to 84 years; and HR 0.99, 95% CI 0.87 to 1.12 for ≥85 years. There was some evidence suggesting that the treatment effect on MACE varied by age (adjusted P value for interaction = 0.050). The diminished relative effects observed in older age groups could be attributed to several factors. These include potentially shorter durations of treatment, a decreased ability to reverse cardiovascular risk as age progresses, and the presence of competing risks for cardiovascular disease. Another consideration is the simple issue of sample size; often, the number of older adults included in these trials is lower, leading to uncertain estimates of treatment effects in this subgroup. Conversely, the absolute risk reductions for MACE demonstrated variation across age groups, showing larger benefits in older populations (adjusted P value for interaction = 0.024). This pattern is likely explained by the higher

Table 1
Randomized, controlled trials of antihypertensive medications in older adults with hypertension

Trial	Date	Achieved BP Intervention	Achieved BP Comparator	Age Criteria	N	Intervention Arm Antihypertensive Medication Regimen	SBP Target Intervention vs comparator[a]	Median Follow-Up (Years)	All-Cause Mortality	MACE	ADE
HYVET[5]	2008	144/78	159/84	≥80 y	3845	TZD ± ACEI	TZD ± ACEI vs placebo	1.8	0.79 (0.65–0.95)	0.66 (0.53–0.82)	358 vs 448 (0.001)
JATOS[17]	2008	136/75	146/78	65–85 y	4418	CCB	<140 vs 140–<160	2	54 vs 42 (0.22)	26 vs 28 (0.78)	NR
bVALISH[16]	2010	137/75	142/77	70–84 y	3260	ARB first line	<140 vs 140–<150	3.1	0.78 (0.46–1.33)	0.84 (0.53–1.36)	281 vs 275 (0.85)
SPRINT-Senior[6]	2016	123/62	135/67	≥75 y	2636	TZD or ACEI/ARB or CCB first line	<120 vs <140	3.1	0.67 (0.49–0.91)	0.66 (0.51–0.85)	0.99 (0.89–1.11)
STEP[7]	2021	127/76	136/79	60–80 y	8511	ARB or CCB first line	110–<130 vs 130–<150	3.3	1.11 (0.78–1.56)	0.72 (0.56–0.93)	Hypotension[c]1.31 (1.02–1.68)

Header note: Intervention vs Comparator (Hazard Ratio [95% CI] or N [P value])

Abbreviations: ACEI, angiotensin-converting enzyme inhibitor; ADE, adverse drug event; AKI, acute kidney injury; ARB, angiotensin-II receptor blocker; BP, blood pressure; CCB, calcium channel blocker; CV, cardiovascular; HYVET, Hypertension in the Very Elderly Trial; JATOS, Japanese trial to assess optimal systolic blood pressure in elderly hypertensive patients; MACE, major adverse cardiovascular event; NR, not reported; SBP, systolic blood pressure; SPRINT, Systolic Blood Pressure Intervention Trial; STEP, strategy of blood pressure intervention in the elderly hypertensive patients; TZD, thiazidelike or thiazidtype diuretic; VALISH, valsartan in elderly isolated systolic hypertension study.

a Unit of measurement for BP is in mm Hg.
b Inclusion criteria was for only adults with isolated systolic hypertension (SBP > 160 and DBP < 90).
c Other ADEs including renal dysfunction were not significantly different between groups.

baseline cardiovascular risk that accompanies advancing age, making even modest reductions in risk factors more impactful in terms of absolute risk reduction.

Applying the best available RCT evidence of the effect of lowering BP with antihypertensive medication to older adults is challenging for 3 predominant reasons:

- First, RCT populations are not fully representative of the target population. Trial designs that explicitly or implicitly exclude older adults with concurrent health issues result in highly selective trial populations. This selectivity is particularly evident in the exclusion of older adults with multiple health conditions, extensive medication use, frailty, and those residing in nursing homes.[22]
- Second, the outcomes measured in RCTs prioritize cardiovascular disease endpoints. There has only been limited enquiry, aside from the SPRINT trial, about the tolerability and degree to which treatment affects ADEs, daily function, and quality of life.
- Third, BP measurement and titration of antihypertensive therapy in a trial setting is not necessarily replicable in routine clinical care. Availability of routine follow-up, access to clinicians and medical staff, and medical resources for hypertension management are not readily available in a real-world context within the current health care landscape.

ANTIHYPERTENSIVE PHARMACOTHERAPY AND ADVERSE DRUG EVENTS IN OLDER ADULTS

A systematic review of 58 RCTs found evidence that antihypertensive medication is associated with acute kidney injury (AKI) with a relative risk (RR) 1.18, 95% CI 1.01 to 1.39; hyperkalemia RR 1.89, 95% CI 1.56 to 2.30; hypotension RR 1.97, 95% CI 1.67 to 2.32; and syncope RR 1.28, 95% CI 1.03 to 1.59, but no evidence of an association with falls RR 1.05, 95% CI 0.89 to 1.24 or fracture RR 0.93, 95% CI 0.58 to 1.48.[23] The lack of individual patient data in this review precluded an analysis of whether treatment effect varied by age. However, it is known that older adults are more susceptible to medication-related ADEs, in part due to altered physiology associated with aging.[24] Older adults undergo many physiological changes which affect drug absorption, distribution, metabolism, and excretion (ADME).[25] **Table 2** provides a review of pharmacokinetic and pharmacodynamic ADME medication changes in older adults.

In an observational study including 3.8 million patients in England aged ≥40 years with hypertension followed up over 10 years,[26] new antihypertensive medication use was associated with an increased risk of hospitalization or death from falls with a HR 1.23, 95% CI 1.21 to 1.26; hypotension HR 1.32, 95% CI 1.29 to 1.35; syncope HR 1.20, 95% CI 1.17 to 1.22; AKI HR 1.44, 95% CI 1.41 to 1.47; electrolyte abnormalities HR 1.45, 95% CI 1.43 to 1.48; and a primary care visit with gout HR 1.35, 95% CI 1.32 to 1.37. Risks of ADEs rose with increasing age and frailty. The robustness of this observational analysis was tested by comparing the results to published estimates from the meta-analysis of RCTs cited earlier[21] and found that the estimates of treatment effect fell within the 95% CIs of estimates from the meta-analysis of RCTs for all outcomes except hypotension and AKI.

GUIDELINE-DIRECTED ANTIHYPERTENSIVE PHARMACOTHERAPY IN OLDER ADULTS

There are 11 classes of antihypertensive medications approved for BP lowering by the US Food and Drug Administration including alpha-blockers, alpha-receptor agonists, beta-blockers, peripheral adrenergic inhibitors, angiotensin-converting enzyme inhibitor (ACEIs), angiotensin-II receptor blockers (ARBs), direct renin inhibitors,

Table 2
Physiologic changes in pharmacokinetic and pharmacodynamic properties of antihypertensive medications associated with aging

Pharmacokinetic/ Pharmacodynamic Property	Definition	Aging-related Changes
Absorption	Absorption of medication into systemic circulation from site of delivery (bioavailability)	1. Decreased gastric acid production, gastric motility, and small bowel surface area resulting in lower medication plasma concentrations. 2. Decreased skin hydration and lipophilicity possibly decreasing transdermal medication absorption (ie, clonidine patch)
Distribution	Distribution of medication into the blood stream and tissues	1. Increased body fat and decreased total body water resulting in increased plasma levels of water-soluble drugs and decreased plasma levels of lipophilic medications. 2. Changes in blood proteins which bind to free medication in the blood stream possibly altering free (ie, unbound) plasma concentrations, thereby, increasing or decreasing their effects and potential for toxicity
Metabolism	Breakdown of medication into water-soluble metabolites for elimination	1. Decreased liver mass, liver and splanchnic blood flow, and liver and intestinal enzyme activity resulting in decreased enzymatic transformation of medication before they reach systemic circulation (first-pass metabolism) 2. Decreased liver volume by up to 30% in older adults also reduces phase I metabolism of medications that interact via the cytochrome P450 enzymes
Excretion	Removal of medication or metabolites from the body (usually via the liver or kidney)	1. Decreased blood flow to the liver and the kidneys, and consequently, drugs which largely depend on blood flow for excretion (ie, drugs with a high "extraction ratio" of >0.7) may experience prolonged elimination times and greater risk for toxicity 2. Decreased kidney size, increased tubular fibrosis and atrophy, and reduced glomerular filtration rate due to hypertension or diabetes may increase plasma concentrations of renally excreted medications

From Refs.[24,25,42,43]

Table 3
Novel antihypertensive medications currently in development

Medication	Mechanism of Action
Aldosterone synthetase inhibitors, for example, lorundrostat, baxdrostat	Blocks the synthesis of aldosterone and thereby prevents aldosterone-mediated sodium and water retention; increases in blood volume and elevated blood pressure.
Angiotensin receptor neprilysin inhibitor, for example, sacubitril/allisartan	Sacubitril blocks neprilysin, the enzyme responsible for breaking down natriuretic peptides. Prolonging activity of natriuretic peptides promotes vasodilation, natriuresis, and diuresis, thereby reducing blood pressure. Allisartan blocks angiotensin-2 receptors to counteract the accumulation of circulating angiotensin 2 caused by neprilysin inhibition.
Attenuators of hepatic angiotensinogen, for example, zilebesiran	Binds hepatic asialoglycoprotein receptor, preventing the formation of hepatic angiotensinogen and thereby blocking activation of the renin–angiotensin–aldosterone system.
Aminopeptidase A inhibitors, for example, firibastat	Inhibits conversion of angiotensin II to angiotensin III in the brain, thereby increasing diuresis and decreasing vasopressin levels, blood volume, sympathetic tone, and vascular resistance.
Atrial natriuretic peptide (ANP) analogs, for example, NCT03781739	Mimics endogenous ANP and inhibits renin and aldosterone, preventing angiotensin II-induced vasoconstriction.
Dual endothelin antagonists, for example, aprocitentan	Blocks endothelin-1 from binding to endothelin A and B receptors on vascular smooth muscle cells, blocking endothelin-1-mediated vasoconstriction, aldosterone synthesis, and catecholamine release.
Glucagonlike peptide-1 (GLP-1) receptor agonists, for example, tirzepatide	Unknown, but may be related to agonism of GLP-1 effects on natriuresis, direct vasodilation, sympathetic activation, or reductions in extracellular volume.

From Blazek, O. and G.L. Bakris, Novel Therapies on the Horizon of Hypertension Management. Am J Hypertens, 2023. 36(2): p. 73–81.

aldosterone receptor antagonists, calcium channel blockers (CCBs), diuretics, and vasodilators. The potential role of novel antihypertensives currently in development (**Table 3**), in the treatment of hypertension in older adults, is currently unclear.[27]

There are only 4 classes recommended as a first-line therapy to lower BP in older adults given their efficacy at preventing cardiovascular disease in RCTs: ACEIs, ARBs, CCBs, and thiazide-like or thiazide-type diuretics (TZDs; **Table 4**). Beta-1 selective adrenoreceptor antagonists also effectively prevent cardiovascular disease events but

Table 4
Preferred antihypertensive medication classes to treat high blood pressure

	ARB/ACEI	CCB[b]	TZD	β-1 Selective Beta-blockers
Mechanism of action	Prevents angiotensin-II-mediated vasoconstriction, sodium retention, and water retention.	Vasodilatation by blocking Ca channels in vascular smooth muscle cells, limited chronotropic and inotropic effect.	Induce natriuresis and diuresis which reduces circulating blood volume.	Block sympathetic adrenergic transmission, negatively ionotropic and chronotropic.
Role in care	First line	First line	First line	Second-line (lower efficacy for preventing CV events)
Compelling indications	Stroke, heart failure, diabetes mellitus, CKD, stable CHD, postmyocardial infarction, aortic disease	Stable angina	Heart failure	Stable CHD/angina, postmyocardial infarction, HFrEF, atrial fibrillation
Contraindications	Severe bilateral renal artery stenosis History of angioedema with ACEIs.[c]	Severe aortic stenosis	Severe hepatic impairment, hypokalemia, COPD (relative)	Asthma, COPD with significant reversibility, heart block
ADEs in older adults >1%	First-dose hypotension, cough,[a] fatigue.	Pedal edema	Dose-dependent: hyponatremia, hypokalemia, hyperuricemia.	Fatigue, bradycardia, diminished exercise tolerance, impaired hypoglycemia awareness.
<1%	Angioedema,[a] acute kidney injury, hyperkalemia	Fatigue, hypotension	New-onset diabetes, hypercalcemia	New-onset diabetes, sleep disorders.

Risk of orthostatic hypotension	Low risk	Low risk	Low risk	Low risk[a]	Verapamil (severe hypotension and cardiac failure)
Harmful drug–drug interactions	Potassium supplements or potassium-sparing diuretics (hyperkalemia), renin inhibitors		CYP3A4 inhibitors, for example, Macrolide antibiotics. (accentuates effect)	Lithium (reduced lithium clearance).	
Renal impairment	Risk of hyperkalemia in established CKD			Switch to a loop diuretic if renal function <30 mL/min.	

Abbreviations: ACEI, angiotensin-converting enzyme inhibitor; ADE, adverse drug event; AKI, acute kidney injury; ARB, angiotensin receptor blocker; CCB, calcium channel blocker; CHD, coronary heart disease; CKD, chronic kidney disease; COPD, chronic obstructive pulmonary disease; CV, cardiovascular; HFrEF, heart failure with reduced ejection fraction; TZD, thiazide-like or thiazide-type diuretic.

a Low quality evidence.
b Dihydropyridine CCBs are more selective to the vasculature and are commonly used in all age groups.
c Patients with angioedema due to ACEI may trial an ARB 6 weeks after stopping ACEI.
From Refs. [13,34,44]

prevent stroke to a lesser degree than other agents and so are second-line agents unless a compelling indication is present. The remaining classes may be added to individualize regimens according to an individual's comorbidities and compelling indications.

The 2023 UK National Institute for Health and Care Excellence (NICE) guidelines distinctly endorse initial CCBs over TZDs in individuals aged 55 years and above based on cost-effectiveness data and lower variability in BP lowering, a factor linked to heightened cardiovascular risk.[28,29] The 2020 Veterans Affairs/Department of Defense recommends TZDs as the first-line treatment in adults aged ≥65 years based on a meta-analysis demonstrating greatest protection against MACE reduction versus other first-line agents without evidence of increase ADEs.[11,30]

EVIDENCE FOR SPECIFIC CLASSES IN OLDER ADULTS

A clinician's selection of a particular agent may be influenced by factors such as other compelling indications, frailty, renal function, and the likelihood of experiencing ADEs.[31] Each class of antihypertensive medication comes with nuanced and distinct advantages and disadvantages when used in older adults and these are considered in **Table 4**. We provide key factors to consider in initial treatment decisions via the BRACE acronym in **Fig. 2**, standing for Benefit, Risk of harm, Adapt, Cost, and Ease.

TITRATION OF THERAPY IN OLDER ADULTS

Historically, clinical guidelines have recommended the "start low, go slow" approach for initiating antihypertensive medication among persons with advanced age, frailty, and multimorbidity. This approach involves starting one medication class at its lowest dose, increasing the dose slowly according to patient response, then adding another

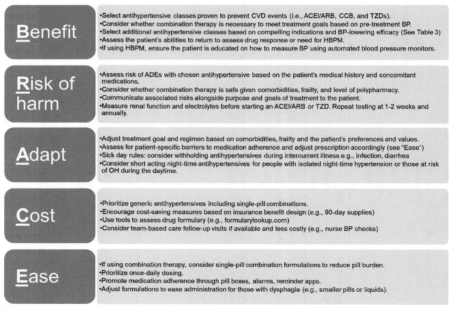

Benefit
- Select antihypertensive classes proven to prevent CVD events (i.e., ACEI/ARB, CCB, and TZDs).
- Consider whether combination therapy is necessary to meet treatment goals based on pre-treatment BP.
- Select additional antihypertensive classes based on compelling indications and BP-lowering efficacy (See Table 3)
- Assess the patient's abilities to return to assess drug response or need for HBPM.
- If using HBPM, ensure the patient is educated on how to measure BP using automated blood pressure monitors.

Risk of harm
- Assess risk of ADEs with chosen antihypertensive based on the patient's medical history and concomitant medications.
- Consider whether combination therapy is safe given comorbidities, frailty, and level of polypharmacy.
- Communicate associated risks alongside purpose and goals of treatment to the patient.
- Measure renal function and electrolytes before starting an ACEI/ARB or TZD. Repeat testing at 1-2 weeks and annually.

Adapt
- Adjust treatment goal and regimen based on comorbidities, frailty and the patient's preferences and values.
- Assess for patient-specific barriers to medication adherence and adjust prescription accordingly (see "Ease")
- Sick day rules: consider withholding antihypertensives during intercurrent illness e.g., infection, diarrhea
- Consider short acting night-time antihypertensives for people with isolated night-time hypertension or those at risk of OH during the daytime.

Cost
- Prioritize generic antihypertensives including single-pill combinations.
- Encourage cost-saving measures based on insurance benefit design (e.g., 90-day supplies)
- Use tools to assess drug formulary (e.g., formularylookup.com)
- Consider team-based care follow-up visits if available and less costly (e.g., nurse BP checks)

Ease
- If using combination therapy, consider single-pill combination formulations to reduce pill burden.
- Prioritize once-daily dosing.
- Promote medication adherence through pill boxes, alarms, reminder apps.
- Adjust formulations to ease administration for those with dysphagia (e.g., smaller pills or liquids).

Fig. 2. BRACE acronym to guide antihypertensive treatment selections for the older adult. ACEI, angiotensin-converting enzyme inhibitor; ADE, adverse drug event; ARB, angiotensin-II receptor blocker; BP, blood pressure; CCB, calcium channel blocker; CVD, cardiovascular disease; TZD, thiazidelike or thiazidetype diuretic.

medication class at its lowest dose, increasing its dose slowly, and so on. This approach requires frequent patient follow-up to assess response and to titrate treatment, and the stepped care approach may increase therapeutic inertia, whereby one medication is initiated and remains unchanged thereafter despite evidence of ineffectiveness.[13] Guidance is lacking on which practice is best for initiating and titrating therapy in older adults, including establishing specific thresholds to determine whether to use mono- or combination therapy.

Considerations on titrating therapy in older adults include

- The risk of first-dose hypotension and highest incidence of ADEs including falls presents in the first 1 to 2 weeks after starting treatment.[32] A large case crossover study demonstrated increased risk of a serious fall injury after initiating an antihypertensive medication, odds ratio (OR) 1.36, 95% CI 1.19 to 1.55, adding a new class, and titration but these associations were not sustained beyond 15 days.[33]
- The requirement to measure standing BP and postural difference in BP to screen for orthostatic hypotension which may be exacerbated by certain classes of antihypertensives more than others.[34] The 2017 American College of Cardiology/American Heart Association hypertension guideline also recommends screening for orthostatic hypotension in people during follow-up after initiation and in higher risk groups (eg, Parkinson's disease and diabetes mellitus).[9]
- The need to check renal function and electrolytes at 1 to 2 weeks and annually thereafter in all first-line antihypertensive classes with the exception of CCBs, but also in the event of intercurrent illness which may increase the risk of electrolyte disturbance or renal failure and indicate the need for a short-term temporary pause of antihypertensive therapy until recovery.[12]

COMBINATION ANTIHYPERTENSIVE PHARMACOTHERAPY IN OLDER ADULTS

Two medication classes each operating through different mechanisms initiated at low doses are more effective and tolerable than monotherapy initiated at standard or maximum doses.[35,36] In younger patients, if the patient's pretreatment SBP is $\geq$20 mm Hg (or DBP is $\geq$10 mm Hg) from their treatment goal, initiation of treatment using combination therapy may be indicated.[9,13] There is uncertainty regarding the relative balance of effectiveness and safety of initiating monotherapy or combination therapy among older adults. Titration of therapy in the context of ADEs may be more difficult if these medications are started in combination rather than individually.

TAILORING ANTIHYPERTENSIVE PHARMACOTHERAPY IN OLDER ADULTS

Hypertension guidelines recommend shared decision-making which is an exercise in empowering a patient to be an agent in their medical care. The 2023 NICE hypertension guidelines offer a decision aid which may help older adults and their caregivers decide whether treatment is feasible for their situation.[12] We recommend considerations relevant to the engagement of older adults in shared decision-making in relation to hypertension treatment (**Fig. 3**).

Presenting risk in terms of absolute risk differences has been shown to be better understood by patients and clinicians.[37] Numbers needed to treat (NNTs) to prevent cardiovascular disease and numbers needed to harm (NNHs) represent an alternative means of presenting benefit and harm to communicate with patients to support shared decision-making about BP treatment. In **Table 5**, the NNT over 5 years has been calculated for different cardiovascular outcomes using data from an IPD meta-analysis of RCTs,[21] alongside NNH over 5 years using data from a large routine

- Invite caregivers to attend, particularly to support patients with fluctuating mental capacity
- Ideally meet more than once, give time for questions
- Provide take-away information to give time to the patient and their family to discuss

- Consider presenting treatment benefit and harm in terms of absolute risk reduction or numbers needed to treat or harm

- Use prediction tools to identify the person's underlying level of risk
  - Cardiovascular risk tools include: QRISK-3 [38]
  - Falls prediction tools include STRATIFY-FALLS [40]
  - Acute Kidney Injury (AKI) prediction tools include STRATIFY-AKI [41]

- Discuss different treatment options in context of
  - Guideline recommendations
  - Compelling indications (comorbidities)
  - Blood tests and monitoring on follow up
  - Risk of side effects

Fig. 3. Step-by-step guide to shared decision-making in hypertension management in older adults.

Table 5
Numbers needed to treat and numbers needed to harm

Event		MACE	Stroke	Ischemic Heart Disease	Heart Failure	Cardiovascular Death	All-cause Mortality
		Numbers Needed to Treat (NNT) at 5 Years[19]					
Age Categories	65–74 y	38	120	55	100	301	100
	75–84 y	25	86	40	75	55	75
	85+ y	23	40	43	151	86	25

Event		Falls	Hypotension	Syncope	Acute kidney Injury	Electrolyte Abnormality	Gout
		Numbers Needed to Harm (NNH) at 5 Years[24]					
Age categories	60–69 y	400	222	250	100	118	125
	70–79 y	118	111	154	47	61	80
	80–89 y	33	56	167	27	27	105
	90+ y	20	51	69	16	19	95

NNTs were calculated over 5 years, as 1/absolute risk reduction associated with the mean blood pressure reduction using event rates in each category associated with treatment compared to control in data representing approximately 3 years follow-up, multiplied by 1.66 to approximate events over 5 years. NNHs were calculated over 5 years, as 1/absolute risk difference (additional events) using event rates over 5 years associated with a new antihypertensive prescription. Color coding is illustrative and does not represent agreed thresholds: for NNT: red >200; amber 100 to 199; green <100; for NNH: red <100; amber 100 to 199; green >200. MACE, major adverse cardiovascular event.
From Refs.[21,26]

data study.[26] This could be used in discussions with patients to support shared decision-making about BP treatment. It is evident from this comparison that across the whole population, the likelihood of benefit from BP-lowering treatment was high, and the likelihood for experiencing harm was very low. However, the risk of benefit and harm becomes more balanced in older age groups. For example, for adults aged 80 to 89 years, prescription of a new BP-lowering treatment may be just as likely to cause a serious fall, as it would prevent a stroke or heart attack: the NNH for a serious fall over 5 years is estimated at 33,[26] the NNT to prevent a major cardiovascular event over 5 years estimated at 23.[21]

Absolute risk prediction is best understood with knowledge of a person's baseline risk of the outcome. This can be estimated using prediction models. To identify patients who may benefit most from BP lowering, guidelines recommend estimating an individual's cardiovascular risk using validated tools (eg, QRISK3,[38] PREVENT [American Heart Association Predicting Risk of CVD Events][39]). Equivalent tools now exist also for identifying a person's risk of developing ADEs related to antihypertensive therapy, specifically their risk of falls (STRATIFY-Falls)[40] and risk of developing AKI (STRATIFY-AKI).[41,42]

SUMMARY

In contrast to historical practices, there are now strong evidence and guideline recommendations endorsing the use of antihypertensive medications in older adults with hypertension. Employing shared decision-making between the clinician and patient is crucial. This process should involve careful consideration of physiological changes with age, the risk of ADEs, and an individualized assessment of the benefits and harms when deciding to initiate or select specific antihypertensive medication therapy for older adults.

CLINICS CARE POINTS

- Evidence supports the cardiovascular and neurovascular benefits of treating hypertension in older adults.

- Across the whole population, the likelihood of benefit from BP-lowering treatment is high, and the likelihood for experiencing harm is very low. However, the risk of benefit and harm becomes more balanced in older age groups.

- Choice of a particular agent should consider compelling indications, concomitant medications, renal function, and the likelihood of experiencing adverse drug events.

- Employing shared decision-making between the clinician and patient is crucial.

- Presenting risk in terms of absolute risk differences is more easily understood by patients and clinicians and best undertaken with knowledge of a person's baseline risk of the outcome.

- Prediction models are available to identify older adults who are at high risk of cardiovascular disease and equivalent tools now also exist for identifying a person's risk of developing adverse drug events related to antihypertensive therapy.

- We recommend the "start low, go slow" approach for initiating antihypertensive medication among older adults.

DISCLOSURE

The work of Dr O.M. Todd is funded by the UK National Institute for Health and Care Research (NIHR) via an Academic Clinical Lectureship. The work of Dr. M. Knight is funded by the UK NIHR via a Specialized Foundation Programme. The work of Dr. J. Sheppard receives funding from the Wellcome Trust, United Kingdom/Royal Society via a Sir Henry Dale Fellowship (ref: 211182/Z/18/Z), the National Institute for Health and Care Research, United Kingdom (NIHR), and from the British Heart Foundation, United Kingdom (refs: PG/21/10,341; FS/19/13/34,235). The work of Dr. A.P. Bress is supported by R01AG74989, K24AG080168, and R01AG065805 from the National Institute on Aging, United States (Bethesda, MD) and R01HL139837 from the National Heart, Lung, and Blood Institute, United States (Bethesda, MD). This research was funded in part by the Wellcome Trust [211182/Z/18/Z]. For the purpose of open access, the author has applied a CC BY public copyright license to any Author Accepted Manuscript version arising from this submission.

REFERENCES

1. Chen V, Ning H, Allen N, et al. Lifetime risks for hypertension by contemporary guidelines in african american and white men and women. JAMA Cardiol 2019; 4(5):455–9.
2. Global Cardiovascular Risk C, Magnussen C, Ojeda FM, et al. Global effect of modifiable risk factors on cardiovascular disease and mortality. N Engl J Med 2023;389(14):1273–85.
3. Rahimi K, Emdin CA, MacMahon S. The epidemiology of blood pressure and its worldwide management. Circ Res 2015;116(6):925–36.
4. World health organisation (WHO). 2023 18.02.2024; Available at: https:// www.who.int/news-room/fact-sheets/detail/cardiovascular-diseases-(cvds)
5. Beckett NS, Peters R, Fletcher AE, et al. Treatment of hypertension in patients 80 years of age or older. N Engl J Med 2008;358(18):1887–98.
6. Williamson JD, Supiano MA, Applegate WB, et al. Intensive vs standard blood pressure control and cardiovascular disease outcomes in adults aged >/=75 years: a randomized clinical trial. JAMA 2016;315(24):2673–82.
7. Zhang W, Zhang S, Deng Y, et al. Trial of intensive blood-pressure control in older patients with hypertension. N Engl J Med 2021;385(14):1268–79.
8. Gabb GM, Mangoni AA, Anderson CS, et al. Guideline for the diagnosis and management of hypertension in adults - 2016. Med J Aust 2016;205(2):85–9.
9. Whelton PK, Carey RM, Aronow WS, et al. 2017 ACC/AHA/AAPA/ABC/ACPM/ AGS/APhA/ASH/ASPC/NMA/PCNA Guideline for the prevention, detection, evaluation, and management of high blood pressure in adults: executive summary: a report of the american college of cardiology/american heart association task force on clinical practice guidelines. Circulation 2018;138(17):e426–83.
10. Rabi DM, McBrien KA, Sapir-Pichhadze R, et al. Hypertension Canada's 2020 comprehensive guidelines for the prevention, diagnosis, risk assessment, and treatment of hypertension in adults and children. Can J Cardiol 2020;36(5): 596–624.
11. Tschanz CMP, Cushman WC, Harrell CTE, et al. Synopsis of the 2020 U.S. department of veterans affairs/u.s. department of defense clinical practice guideline: the diagnosis and management of hypertension in the primary care setting. Ann Intern Med 2020;173(11):904–13.
12. (NICE). N.I.f.H.a.C.E. Hypertension in adults: diagnosis and management. 2023 18.02.2024. Available at: http://www.ncbi.nlm.nih.gov/books/NBK547161/.
13. Mancia G, Kreutz R, Brunström M, et al. 2023 ESH guidelines for the management of arterial hypertension the task force for the management of arterial hypertension of the european society of hypertension: endorsed by the international

society of hypertension (ISH) and the European renal association (ERA). J Hypertens 2023;41(12):1874–2071.

14. Qaseem A, Wilt TJ, Rich R, et al. Pharmacologic treatment of hypertension in adults aged 60 years or older to higher versus lower blood pressure targets: a clinical practice guideline from the American college of physicians and the american academy of family physicians. Ann Intern Med 2017;166(6):430–7.

15. Bogaerts JMK, von Ballmoos LM, Achterberg WP, et al. Do we AGREE on the targets of antihypertensive drug treatment in older adults: a systematic review of guidelines on primary prevention of cardiovascular diseases. Age Ageing 2022;51(1):afab192.

16. Ogihara T, Saruta T, Rakugi H, et al. Target blood pressure for treatment of isolated systolic hypertension in the elderly: valsartan in elderly isolated systolic hypertension study. Hypertension 2010;56(2):196–202.

17. Group JS. Principal results of the Japanese trial to assess optimal systolic blood pressure in elderly hypertensive patients (JATOS). Hypertens Res 2008;31(12): 2115–27.

18. Warwick J, Falaschetti E, Rockwood K, et al. No evidence that frailty modifies the positive impact of antihypertensive treatment in very elderly people: an investigation of the impact of frailty upon treatment effect in the HYpertension in the Very Elderly Trial (HYVET) study, a double-blind, placebo-controlled study of antihypertensives in people with hypertension aged 80 and over. BMC Med 2015; 13:78.

19. Wang Z, Du X, Hua C, et al. The effect of frailty on the efficacy and safety of intensive blood pressure control: a post hoc analysis of the SPRINT trial. Circulation 2023;148(7):565–74.

20. Sheppard JP, Lown M, Burt J, et al. Generalizability of blood pressure lowering trials to older patients: cross-sectional analysis. J Am Geriatr Soc 2020;68(11): 2508–15.

21. Blood Pressure Lowering Treatment TrialistsC.. Age-stratified and blood-pressure-stratified effects of blood-pressure-lowering pharmacotherapy for the prevention of cardiovascular disease and death: an individual participant-level data meta-analysis. Lancet 2021;398(10305):1053–64.

22. He J, Morales DR, Guthrie B. Exclusion rates in randomized controlled trials of treatments for physical conditions: a systematic review. Trials 2020;21(1):228.

23. Albasri A, Hattle M, Koshiaris C, et al. Association between antihypertensive treatment and adverse events: systematic review and meta-analysis. BMJ 2021;372:n189.

24. Mangoni AA, Jackson SH. Age-related changes in pharmacokinetics and pharmacodynamics: basic principles and practical applications. Br J Clin Pharmacol 2004;57(1):6–14.

25. Drenth-van Maanen AC, Wilting I, Jansen PAF. Prescribing medicines to older people-How to consider the impact of ageing on human organ and body functions. Br J Clin Pharmacol 2020;86(10):1921–30.

26. Sheppard JP, Koshiaris C, Stevens R, et al. The association between antihypertensive treatment and serious adverse events by age and frailty: a cohort study. PLoS Med 2023;20(4):e1004223.

27. Blazek O, Bakris GL. Novel therapies on the horizon of hypertension management. Am J Hypertens 2023;36(2):73–81.

28. (UK), N.C.G.C. Hypertension: The clinical management of primary hypertension in adults: update of clinical guidelines 18 and 34. 2011 18.02.2024. Available at: http://www.ncbi.nlm.nih.gov/books/NBK83274/.

29. Webb AJ, Fischer U, Mehta Z, et al. Effects of antihypertensive-drug class on interindividual variation in blood pressure and risk of stroke: a systematic review and meta-analysis. Lancet 2010;375(9718):906–15.
30. Thomopoulos C, Parati G, Zanchetti A. Effects of blood pressure-lowering treatment on cardiovascular outcomes and mortality: 14 - effects of different classes of antihypertensive drugs in older and younger patients: overview and meta-analysis. J Hypertens 2018;36(8):1637–47.
31. Ettehad D, Emdin CA, Kiran A, et al. Blood pressure lowering for prevention of cardiovascular disease and death: a systematic review and meta-analysis. Lancet 2016;387(10022):957–67.
32. Kahlaee HR, Latt MD, Schneider CR. Association between chronic or acute use of antihypertensive class of medications and falls in older adults. a systematic review and meta-analysis. Am J Hypertens 2018;31(4):467–79.
33. Shimbo D, Barrett Bowling C, Levitan EB, et al. Short-term risk of serious fall injuries in older adults initiating and intensifying treatment with antihypertensive medication. Circ Cardiovasc Qual Outcomes 2016;9(3):222–9.
34. Juraschek SP, Cortez MM, Flack JM, et al. Orthostatic hypotension in adults with hypertension: a scientific statement from the american heart association. Hypertension 2024;81(3):e16–30.
35. Wald DS, Law M, Morris JK, et al. Combination therapy versus monotherapy in reducing blood pressure: meta-analysis on 11,000 participants from 42 trials. Am J Med 2009;122(3):290–300.
36. Law MR, Wald NJ, Morris JK, et al. Value of low dose combination treatment with blood pressure lowering drugs: analysis of 354 randomised trials. BMJ 2003; 326(7404):1427.
37. Zipkin DA, Umscheid CA, Keating NL, et al. Evidence-based risk communication: a systematic review. Ann Intern Med 2014;161(4):270–80.
38. Hippisley-Cox J, Coupland C, Brindle P. Development and validation of QRISK3 risk prediction algorithms to estimate future risk of cardiovascular disease: prospective cohort study. BMJ 2017;357:j2099.
39. Khan SS, Coresh J, Pencina MJ, et al. Novel prediction equations for absolute risk assessment of total cardiovascular disease incorporating cardiovascular-kidney-metabolic health: a scientific statement from the american heart association. Circulation 2023;148(24):1982–2004.
40. Archer L, Koshiaris C, Lay-Flurrie S, et al. Development and external validation of a risk prediction model for falls in patients with an indication for antihypertensive treatment: retrospective cohort study. BMJ 2022;379:e070918.
41. Koshiaris C, Archer L, Lay-Flurrie S, et al. Predicting the risk of acute kidney injury in primary care: derivation and validation of STRATIFY-AKI. Br J Gen Pract 2023; 73(733):e605–14.
42. Kaestli LZ, Wasilewski-Rasca AF, Bonnabry P, et al. Use of transdermal drug formulations in the elderly. Drugs Aging 2008;25(4):269–80.
43. Butler JM, Begg EJ. Free drug metabolic clearance in elderly people. Clin Pharmacokinet 2008;47(5):297–321.
44. Bhanu C, Nimmons D, Petersen I, et al. Drug-induced orthostatic hypotension: a systematic review and meta-analysis of randomised controlled trials. PLoS Med 2021;18(11):e1003821.

Resistant Hypertension in Older Adults

John M. Giacona, PhD, PA-C[a,b], Wanpen Vongpatanasin, MD[b,*]

KEYWORDS

- Hypertension • Older adults • Secondary hypertension

KEY POINTS

- Resistant hypertension is highly prevalent in older adults.
- The mainstay lifestyle change is decreasing dietary sodium intake.
- Investigate for secondary causes of hypertension as clinically indicated.

DEFINITION

Resistant hypertension (RHTN) is defined as having uncontrolled blood pressure (BP) despite maximum or maximally tolerated doses of ≥ 3 antihypertensive drugs that includes a long-acting calcium channel blocker (CCB), a renin-angiotensin system (RAS) blocker, and a diuretic.[1,2] Hypertension (HTN) that requires the use of ≥ 4 antihypertensive drugs is also considered as RHTN regardless of BP.[2]

It should be mentioned that the 2017 American College of Cardiology/American Heart Association guideline for the management of high BP defines controlled BP less than 130/80 mm Hg for older adults aged ≥ 65 years, which is a similar BP target for younger adults. However, the recommendation is specific to noninstitutionalized, ambulatory older adults living independently in the community without frequent falls or advanced cognitive impairment that predispose them to increased adverse events from intensive BP lowering.[1]

PREVALENCE

Prevalence of apparent RHTN is estimated to be 16% to 20% in all US adults with treated HTN.[3,4] As expected, it is more common in older adults ≥ 60 years of age (20%–30%) when compared to younger adults 20 to 59 years of age (10%–14%).[4] Aside from older age, black race, male sex, presence of obstructive sleep apnea

[a] Department of Applied Clinical Research, University of Texas Southwestern Medical Center, 5323 Harry Hines Boulevard, H4.130, Dallas, TX 75390-8586, USA; [b] Cardiology Division, Department of Internal Medicine, University of Texas Southwestern Medical Center, 5323 Harry Hines Boulevard, H4.130, Dallas, TX, USA
* Corresponding author.
E-mail address: wanpen.vongpatanasin@utsouthwestern.edu
Twitter: @GiaconaJohn (J.M.G.); @DrWanpen (W.V.)

Clin Geriatr Med 40 (2024) 645–658
https://doi.org/10.1016/j.cger.2024.04.005
0749-0690/24/© 2024 Elsevier Inc. All rights reserved.

(OSA), obesity, heart failure (HF), diabetes mellitus (DM), and chronic kidney disease (CKD) are also risk factors of RHTN.[2,5]

INITIAL APPROACH TO ASSESSMENT AND EVALUATION
Assess for Pseudo-resistance

The recommended first step in evaluating RHTN is to exclude pseudo-resistance. The 2 common causes of pseudo-RHTN are white-coat HTN and patient medication non-adherence. The white-coat BP effect is defined in treated adults as an office BP $\geq$ 130/80 mm Hg with an out-of-office BP that is at or below goal, based on a 24-hour ambulatory BP monitoring of $\leq$ 125/75 mm Hg, or a home BP $\leq$ 130/80 mm Hg. Importantly, a large cohort study found that the white-coat effect was present in about 37.5% of adult patients with RHTN and was associated with older age adults.[6,7] As such, the presence or absence of the white-coat effect should be identified by performing out-of-office BP monitoring prior to diagnosing true RHTN.[8] In addition, nonadherence to medication is highly prevalent in those with RHTN in older adults, which may be related to complex medication regimens, medication side effects, drug costs, or cognitive impairment.[9]

There are many methods to assess medication adherence (eg, pharmacy refill, questionnaires, and self-reports). One emerging technique is the use of therapeutic drug monitoring (TDM). Prior studies have demonstrated greater utility in detecting medication nonadherence using TDM when compared to self-report and pharmacy refill methods.[10,11] If suboptimal adherence to medication use is established, potential barriers causing the nonadherence should be explored, including complexity of regimen, cost, and cognitive deficit. In older adults, focusing on more simplified regimens (eg, once-daily dosing vs medications requiring multiple daily doses, or fixed dose combination pills when available), including reminder methods (eg, using a pill box), and involving family members and caregivers in the treatment plan may aid in increasing medication adherence.

Evaluate for Blood Pressure–Raising Agents

Certain substances shown in **Box 1**, such as illicit drugs and over-the-counter (OTC) or nonprescription medications, can raise BP and should be evaluated prior to making a diagnosis of RHTN. The most common substances used in the general population of adults with HTN in the United States include antidepressants, nonsteroidal anti-inflammatory drugs (NSAIDs), and exogenous steroids, estrogens, and testosterones,[12]

Box 1
Common substances that can raise blood pressure and worsen hypertension that should be evaluated for during initial assessment

Common substances that can raise blood pressure
- Nonsteroidal anti-inflammatory drugs
- Antidepressants
- Exogenous steroids, estrogens, and testosterones
- Stimulants (eg, pseudoephedrine)
- Illicit drugs (eg, cocaine)
- Decongestant (eg, oxymetazoline)
- Glycyrrhetinic acid (licorice root)
- Cyclosporine
- Erythropoietin

while the most used OTC medications in older adults (age >70 years) that may affect BP includes NSAIDs (namely naproxen and aspirin) and acetaminophen.[13]

Evaluation for Secondary Hypertension

An important consideration in older patients with RHTN is the proper screening, awareness of clinical presentation, and identification of secondary causes of HTN. The most common are included in **Table 1**.

Primary aldosteronism (PA): PA is characterized by the inappropriate and autonomous secretion of aldosterone from the adrenal glands which results in suppression of the RAS. PA can be generally categorized as a unilateral (hypersecretion from one adrenal gland) or bilateral (hypersecretion from both adrenal glands) condition. Bilateral PA (sometimes termed "idiopathic hyperaldosteronism") accounts for 60% to 70% cases, making it more common than unilateral PA. Unilateral forms account for the remaining 30% to 40% of cases, and can consist of aldosterone-producing adenomas (APAs), aldosterone-producing diffuse hyperplasia, or hyperplasia with APA, aldosterone-producing nodules, or aldosterone-producing micronodules (APMs).[14] Rarely, PA can present as an aldosterone-producing adrenocortical carcinoma or a familial form of PA.

PA is considered the most common form of endocrine HTN with a 10% to 15% prevalence among stage I HTN and a 20% to 30% prevalence among adults with treatment RHTN.[14] While prior evidence suggests there may be a decreased prevalence of overt PA with age (especially in adults ≥70 years),[15] recent evidence has demonstrated that a progressive accumulation of APMs occurs with aging.[14] The age-dependent accumulation of APMs may explain increased salt sensitivity with aging/in older adults.[16]

Screening for PA includes assessment of plasma renin activity (PRA) and plasma aldosterone concentration (PAC). These tests can be initially performed during treatment with mineralocorticoid receptor antagonists (MRAs) or other RAS blockade medications.[14] Positive screening is a suppressed PRA (<1.0 ng/ml/h) in patients considered to be high risk, regardless of the medication use at the time of screening. Importantly, a suppressed PRA while taking MRAs, other RAS blockade medications, direct renin inhibitors, thiazides, or thiazidelike diuretics during the time of screening should increase the clinician's suspicion for PA, as these typically increase PRA. It's important to note that the absence of hypokalemia does not preclude the possibility of PA as only 20% to 50% of PA patients present with hypokalemia.[17]

If the patient is on MRA therapy, other RAS blockade medications, or any of the agents that may interfere with screening such as direct renin inhibitors, thiazides, or thiazidelike diuretics, and PRA is not suppressed despite high clinical suspicion for PA, it's advisable to repeat PA screening in more optimal conditions.[14] Specifically, a 2-week washout period from thiazides, angiotensin-converting enzyme inhibitors (ACEIs), or angiotensin receptor blockers (ARBs); a 4-week washout period from MRAs; and (if present) normalization of hypokalemia (with serum potassium goal 4.0–5.0 mmol/L) are recommended prior to the repeat screening to avoid a false-negative result.[18] Medications that patients can be switched to during this time that are known to have minimal effects on the renin-angiotensin-aldosterone system (RAAS) include CCBs, hydralazine, or alpha-adrenergic receptor blockers (α-AR blockers). In the presence of suppressed PRA, an elevated PAC (≥10 ng/dL) strongly suggests the presence of PA. If PA is suspected to be present, referral to HTN specialists for additional confirmatory testing (ie, salt loading test), lateralization (ie, adrenal vein sampling (AVS)), and continued HTN treatment is recommended.

Pheochromocytomas: Pheochromocytomas and paragangliomas (PGLs) are rare neuroendocrine tumors that cause excess production and secretion of catecholamines.

Table 1
Common causes of secondary hypertension and associated screening and confirmatory testing recommendations

Cause of Secondary Hypertension	Clinical Indication	Initial Screening Test(s)	Confirmatory/Diagnostic Test(s)
Primary aldosteronism	Severe or resistant HTN HTN with unexplained or diuretic-induced hypokalemia, adrenal mass, atrial fibrillation, or OSA	Plasma renin activity and aldosterone levels during optimal conditions (serum potassium of 4.0–5.0 mmol/L and withdrawal of all aldosterone antagonists for > 4 wk)	Oral salt loading test (with 24-h urine aldosterone) Adrenal CT scan Adrenal vein sampling
OSA	Resistant HTN with snoring, witnessed breathing pauses during sleep, or excessive daytime sleepiness/fatigue	Berlin Questionnaire Overnight oximetry	Polysomnography
Renovascular disease	Atherosclerotic renal artery stenosis: Resistant HTN Short-onset severe HTN Acutely worsening or increasingly difficult to control HTN Fibromuscular dysplasia: Early-onset HTN, especially in women	Renal duplex Doppler ultrasound Abdominal CT	CT or magnetic resonance angiogram of renal arteries

Abbreviations: CT, computed tomography; HTN, hypertension; OSA, obstructive sleep apnea.

pheochromocytomas and PGLs (PPGLs) have an estimated prevalence of 0.01% to 0.2%, with a higher prevalence of ~4% in those presenting with RHTN.[2] Though most cases are sporadic, it's estimated that 30% to 40% of cases are genetically inherited. Major familial disorders associated with pheochromocytomas include von Hippel-Lindau, multiple endocrine neoplasia type 2A and 2B, and neurofibromatosis.

Generally, pheochromocytomas are diagnosed in the fourth and fifth decades of life and are rare in older adults. However, they can be either benign or metastatic. Though malignancy is rare for adrenal pheochromocytomas (around 10% are metastatic), PGLs carry a much higher frequency of malignancy around 30% to 70%. The common "classical" symptoms of PPGLs include sustained HTN, and/or labile hypertensive episodes accompanied by headache, anxiety, palpitations or tachycardia, and pallor. Another presentation is orthostatic hypotension that is common with tumors that predominantly secrete epinephrine due to β-2 adrenergic receptor–mediated vasodilation.

Specific biochemical testing recommended includes measurements of plasma free metanephrines or urinary fractionated metanephrines, as they have been shown to be more sensitive than other tests of catecholamine excess for the diagnosis of PPGLs (ie, plasma or urinary catecholamines, or urinary vanillylmandelic acid).[19] Elevation of plasma or urinary metanephrines of $\geq$ 4 times above the upper limit of normal (based on laboratory reference standard) can be considered diagnostic for pheochromocytomas. On the other hand, having normal level of plasma free metanephrines generally excludes the presence of pheochromocytomas. Borderline elevations (below 4 times the upper limit of normal) could represent sympathetic overactivity, which is a common feature in patients with HTN, obesity, or particularly OSA.

Once there is positive biochemical evidence of a PPGL, imaging studies to locate the PPGLs should be pursued which include computed tomography (CT) or magnetic resonance imaging (MRI) of the abdomen and pelvis. For the head and neck region, MRI is preferred over CT due to MRI having high sensitivity (90% and 95%), while for detecting potential lung metastases, CT is preferred over MRI. Recent evidence suggests that positron emission tomography (PET)/CT utilizing gallium-68 DOTATATE is superior to meta-iodobenzylguanidine scintigraphy in detecting most metastatic PPGLs and should be considered the tracer of choice in this setting.[20] PET/CT with fluorodopa F[18] study may be useful in some PGL patients with succinate dehydrogenase subunit D mutation.

Cushing's syndrome (CS): CS is an uncommon endocrine form of HTN, accounting for less than 1% of hypertensive patients. CS is caused by the chronic and excessive exposure to endogenous or exogenous glucocorticoids. Excessive exposure to glucocorticoids may be the results of oversecretion of adrenocorticotropin hormone (ACTH; ACTH-dependent), or excessive circulating levels of glucocorticoids (ACTH-independent). The most common cause of CS is exogenous glucocorticoids, while Cushing's disease (CD) is the most common cause of endogenous CS (identified in 70% of patients) and is due to an ACTH-secreting pituitary tumor. Others include ectopic ACTH syndrome, adrenal adenoma, adrenal carcinoma, or adrenal hyperplasia, but are much less common and account for about 10% to 15% of cases.

The more classical signs include truncal obesity, purplish abdominal striae, easy bruising, facial flushing, and a dorsocervical fat pad ("buffalo hump"). However, among older adults of age greater than 60 years, observational evidence suggests that CD typically presents with more catabolic characteristics, such as having lower body mass index (despite greater central adiposity), greater prevalence of muscle wasting, and less hirsutism among women.[21] Moreover, older adults had higher prevalence of comorbidities, namely HTN and DM.

The screening and diagnosis of CS should begin by evaluating the cortisol secretory status of the patient with one of the tests listed in **Table 2**, and abnormalities in at least 2 screening tests are needed before the diagnosis of CS can be confirmed.[22]

Once CS is diagnosed as described earlier, the next step is to delineate if the CS is an ACTH-dependent or ACTH-independent form. Plasma ACTH should be obtained at 8 AM to separate ACTH-dependent forms from ACTH-independent forms of CS. Plasma ACTH concentrations below 5 pg/mL (1.1 pmol/L) at 8 AM indicates the presence of ACTH-independent disease, whereas plasma levels above 10 (2.2 pmol/L) suggests the presence of ACTH-dependent CS. Patients with ACTH-independent CS should undergo adrenal imaging by CT or MRI, while patients with ACTH-dependent CS should undergo pituitary imaging and tumor localization by MRI. For patients with ACTH-dependent CS, if pituitary MRI fails to detect a tumor, the next step includes inferior petrosal sinus sampling to differentiate the presence of small pituitary tumors from an ectopic (non-pituitary) ACTH-producing tumor.

OSA: Screening for sleep disorders should be considered in RHTN patients with high clinical suspicion. Specifically, OSA is highly prevalent among patients with RHTN, with rates up to 70% to 90%. Established risk factors for OSA include adults of older age, male sex, and the presence of PA, and obesity.[2] The mechanisms underlying OSA contribution to elevated BP are multifactorial and include overactivation of the sympathetic nervous system and the RAS from chronic nighttime hypoxemia.[23]

Table 2 Summary of diagnostic tests for Cushing's syndrome	
Test/Method/Interpretation	**Comments**
Late night salivary cortisol test (LNSC): Salivary samples on 2–3 different nights are collected between 11 PM and 12 AM. Samples are stable in room temperature for several days. The criteria used to interpret salivary cortisol results differ due to assay differences. Follow specific laboratory reference ranges.	*Advantages:* Recommended in cyclic Cushing's syndrome and adrenal incidentaloma. Noninvasive and can be easily performed at home. *Disadvantages:* Not reliable in night shift workers, smokers, and patients who use licorice or chew tobacco.
1-mg dexamethasone suppression test (DST): A 1-mg dose of oral dexamethasone is administered between 11 PM and 12 AM prior to sample collection. Serum cortisol is measured between 8 AM and 9 AM the next morning. Cortisol level of > 1.8 μg/dL at 8 AM is suggestive of Cushing's syndrome.	*Advantages:* More sensitive than urinary free cortisol in patients with adrenal incidentaloma. Preferred test for shift workers and patients with disrupted circadian rhythm due to uneven sleep schedules. *Disadvantages:* Certain medications can affect absorption and metabolism of dexamethasone by induction or inhibition of cytochrome P450 3A4. Conditions that increase cortisol-binding globulin may falsely elevate cortisol levels (eg, taking oral estrogens).
24-h urinary free cortisol (UFC): 24-h urine specimens (considered appropriate using total volume and creatinine concentration) should be collected at least 2–3 times. Values above the upper limit of normal are suspicious for Cushing's syndrome.	*Advantages:* Not affected by levels of cortisol-binding globulin. *Disadvantages:* Results unreliable in renal failure patients and in patients with high fluid intake (>5 L/d).

Patients with OSA will typically present with loud snoring, witnessed apneas during sleep, and episodes of gasping or choking during the night. Patients may also report daytime sleepiness, drowsiness, or general fatigue, or involuntary periods of dozing. Indications for OSA screening include resistant or poorly controlled HTN, recurrent atrial fibrillation (after previous ablation or cardioversion), and pulmonary HTN. Once OSA is suspected, patients should undergo one of the following tests for screening: the Berlin Questionnaire, the STOP-BANG (snoring, tiredness, observed apnea, blood pressure, body mass index, age, neck circumference, and gender), or overnight oximetry. For diagnosis, patients should undergo either an overnight in-laboratory, multichannel polysomnography or a home sleep apnea test.[23]

Renal parenchymal disease: CKD is one of the most common causes of secondary HTN and therefore should be viewed as both a complication and a cause of suboptimal BP control. Importantly, CKD is well known to be an age-related condition with a 40% "lifetime risk" of developing CKD in older adults.[2,24] Pathophysiological mechanisms of CKD that may worsen BP control include reductions in renal function resulting in suboptimal sodium and water excretion (eg, volume overload), overactivation of the RAAS, and elevated sympathetic nervous system discharge.

Diagnosis and evaluation of renal impairment includes obtaining serum creatinine, cystatin C, and urine albumin-creatinine ratio to adequately assess the stage and prognosis of CKD. Serum cystatin C is less affected by muscle mass, age, or sex, when compared with creatinine and is currently recommended to confirm estimated glomerular filtration rate (eGFR) in adults who are at risk for or have CKD.[25,26] Ultrasonography should be considered to determine kidney size and exclude adult polycystic kidney disease.

Renovascular HTN: Renovascular HTN is a very common cause of RHTN in older adults.[2] Atherosclerotic renal artery stenosis (ARAS) and fibromuscular dysplasia (FMD) are both subtypes of renovascular disease, but ARAS is much more prevalent among older adults. Specifically, data suggest that 24% of adults of age greater than 70 years with RHTN have significant ARAS, while FMD is more common in younger women. Much less common causes of renal artery obstruction include Takayasu's arteritis, radiation fibrosis, or renal artery dissection. ARAS can range from an asymptomatic finding to renal insufficiency with accelerated or malignant HTN. Pathophysiological mechanisms related to suboptimal BP control in ARAS stem from renal hypoperfusion due to the atherosclerotic obstruction, which results in subsequent reflex activation of RAAS that causes sodium and fluid retention.

ARAS or FMD can initially by investigated with the use of renal duplex Doppler ultrasonography aimed at determining peak systolic velocity (PSV) in the renal arteries and the renal-to-aortic ratio (RAR).[2] The presence of renal artery PSV of $\geq$ 180 cm/sec and an RAR $\geq$ 3.5 indicates severe stenosis.[27] Duplex Doppler can then be followed by more sensitive imaging studies such as CT or magnetic resonance angiography of the renal arteries. Imaging will also inform the clinician if unilateral or bilateral ARAS is present, which can help guide future medical decision-making.

MANAGEMENT AND TREATMENT
Implement and Reinforce Lifestyle Modifications

There is consistent evidence supporting the benefit of sodium restriction in RHTN.[28,29] As such, recent guidelines recommend reducing dietary sodium intake to less than 1500 mg per day as a mainstay in nonpharmacologic treatment.[1]

In addition to dietary changes, increasing physical activity has been recognized as an effective lifestyle modification to reduce BP in patients with RHTN. Patients of all ages with RHTN can achieve significant reductions in BP through incorporating 120 minutes per week of moderate intensity aerobic exercise training (eg, walking).[30] In older adults $\geq$ 60 years of age, moderate intensity anaerobic or resistance training (eg, using free weights) has also been shown to reduce BP in those with HTN.[31] As such, older adults have several methods to increase exercise that can be tailored to their current ability and preference.

Treatment of Secondary Hypertension

For secondary HTN, therapy should be directed at the specific causes. Patients who are suspected to have endocrine HTN (PA, PGLs or pheochromocytomas, or CS) should be referred to endocrinologists or HTN specialists who are familiar with management of the specific endocrine disorders. Likewise, patients with sleep disorders (such as OSA) should be referred and evaluated by sleep medicine specialists. Patients with renovascular HTN should be referred to HTN specialists and vascular medicine/surgery for comanagement.

PA: The approach to management of PA largely depends on whether aldosterone overproduction is unilateral or bilateral. In patients with bilateral PA, or those with unilateral PA, who do not desire surgery or are too frail to undergo surgery, the recommended treatment is with MRAs and dietary sodium restriction (<1500 mg per day). It should be noted that higher doses of spironolactone (up to 225 mg daily) or eplerenone (up to 300 mg/day) may be needed to adequately control BP and accomplish PRA supression,[32] and that sodium restriction can have significant impact in the normalization of BP and raise renin in those with PA.[33] Surgical adrenalectomy should be offered for patients with unilateral type PA (ie, those who have a lateralization index $\geq$ 4 on AVS), as it has been shown to resolve HTN in 10% to 20% of patients.[34]

Pheochromocytoma: Surgical treatment is the mainstay therapy for patients with PPGL. Importantly, all patients should receive preoperative treatment for 7 to 14 days with a nonselective α-adrenergic receptor (AR) blocker (eg, phenoxybenzamine) or an α_1-selective AR blocker (eg, doxazosin) to block vasoconstriction related to the potential release of catecholamines during intraoperative manipulation of the tumors. If further BP control is required, CCBs (eg, amlodipine or nifedipine) are recommended as the add-on drug class.[35] Treatment with β-AR blockers to prevent tachycardia should be initiated only after the development of reflex tachycardia from the use of α-AR blockers. Due to the risk of potential hypertensive crisis from unopposed stimulation of α-adrenergic receptors, the use of β-AR blockers first, as monotherapy (ie, in the absence of an α-AR blocker), is not recommended. For patients with metastatic diseases, surgical debulking of the primary tumor is also recommended to minimize catecholamine release and morbidity associated with catecholamine excess.

CS: The first-line and mainstay treatment for CS caused by adrenal or pituitary tumors is surgical resection of the primary lesion(s), unless surgery is not possible (eg, patient would not like to pursue or they are too frail), or if the surgery is unlikely to significantly reduce the glucocorticoid excess. As such, patients with pituitary tumors should be referred to adrenal and/or pituitary surgeons with extensive experience with these procedures.

The second-line options for those with ACTH-dependent CS should be chosen in a shared decision-making approach with an experienced endocrinologist. These options include repeating the transsphenoidal surgery, initiating pituitary-directed medications, or radiation therapy (this carries a risk of hypopituitarism). Medical therapy as a second-line option is recommended after transsphenoidal surgery in patients with CD, as primary treatment of ectopic ACTH secretion in patients with metastases, and as adjunct therapy in adrenocortical carcinoma to reduce cortisol levels.[36] Examples of medical therapy includes using adrenal steroidogenesis inhibitors (eg, osilodrostat), targeting pituitary somatostatin and dopamine receptors (eg, the dopamine agonist cabergoline), and targeting peripheral glucocorticoid receptors (eg, the glucocorticoid receptor blocker mifepristone).

OSA: There are several treatment options for OSA, some of which include continuous positive airway pressure (PAP) (CPAP), auto-titrating PAP, bilevel PAP, oral appliances, upper airway surgery or hypoglossal nerve stimulation (HGNS), lifestyle intervention/medical weight loss, and bariatric surgery. For patients with RHTN, a previous meta-analysis of clinical trials demonstrated that treatment of OSA with CPAP is associated with 5 mm Hg reductions in 24-hour ambulatory systolic BP (SBP), with greater reductions in BP observed among patients with long-term adherence to CPAP therapy ($\geq$4 h/day).[37] Aside from the observed improvements in BP control, clinical trials incorporating CPAP have also shown improvements in patient-reported sleepiness, drowsiness, and overall quality of life. HGNS has been shown to reduce apnea hypopnea index and approved for the treatment of OSA. However, a randomized sham-controlled clinical trial showed no effect of HGNS on 24-hour ambulatory BP.[38] Newer approaches to stimulate the proximal portion of the nerve may increase effectiveness in reducing airway obstruction and BP than distal nerve stimulation used in earlier trials.[39]

Renovascular disease: The mainstay of treatment for moderately severe unilateral ARAS consists of blocking the RAS with the use of ACEIs/ARBs.[2] Importantly, evidence suggests that most patients can tolerate ACEIs/ARBs without adverse renal effects. However, 10% to 20% may not tolerate ACEIs/ARBs due to increases in serum creatinine following medication initiation. However, these patients can typically tolerate restarting the ACEIs/ARBs after successful revascularization (if this becomes a reasonable treatment choice). Thus, close monitoring of renal function is warranted when starting or increasing the dose of these medications.

Renal artery angioplasty should be considered for all RHTN patients with FMD. However, the role of renal stenting in ARAS remains controversial. Although previous randomized controlled trials in HTN patients with ARAS showed a small benefit of renal artery stenting on BP with no improvement in cardiovascular or renal outcomes,[40] subsequent observational studies suggest greater benefit among RHTN patients, and in selected subgroups of patients with younger age or new-onset HTN (<1 y) without proteinuria.[41] Renal stenting should also be considered for severe bilateral renal artery stenosis or stenosis of a solitary native kidney, as pharmacotherapy plays a more limited role.

Optimize Pharmacotherapy

The optimal 3-drug regimen for RHTN should include an ACEI or ARB, a CCB, and a thiazide or thiazidelike diuretic, titrated to maximal or maximally tolerated doses.[1,2] Choice of the appropriate diuretic based on renal function is crucial for the successful management of BP in RHTN. Thus, after the 3-drug regimen has been titrated appropriately, consider optimizing the patient's diuretic therapy by switching the current diuretic to chlorthalidone (CTD), with the exception for patients with end-stage CKD (eGFR less than 15 mL/min1.73 m^2), or on those on dialysis. Recent evidence from a randomized trial demonstrated that in patients with stage-IV CKD and uncontrolled HTN, CTD treatment for 3 months significantly reduced 24-hour BP by 11/4 mm Hg when compared with placebo.[42] For patients who have severely reduced renal function, consideration of a long-acting loop diuretic such as torsemide is recommended.

MRAs, such as spironolactone, should be considered as the fourth-line medication (for eGFR > 30 mL/min1.73 m^2). Supporting randomized clinical trial evidence demonstrated spironolactone to be superior to an α-AR blocker and β-AR blockers in reducing BP in patients with RHTN.[43] However, spironolactone at high doses in men can often result in gynecomastia and erectile dysfunction, which may limit its use. In these cases, eplerenone[2] or amiloride[44] can be used as suitable alternatives.

The decision on the next agent may be informed by patient characteristics, such as the existence of comorbidities (eg, DM, HF, CKD), or through assessment of sympathetic tone (ie, resting heart rate (HR)). For patients with RHTN and DM or CKD, the addition of a sodium-glucose cotransport 2 inhibitor may offer BP lowering in addition at cardiorenal protection.[45] Recently, a post hoc analysis of PARAGON-HF (Efficacy and Safety of LCZ696 Compared to Valsartan, on Morbidity and Mortality in Heart Failure Patients With Preserved Ejection Fraction) trial data demonstrated that the combination of sacubitril-valsartan significantly reduced BP compared to valsartan alone in older patients (>70 years) with HF and preserved ejection fraction and apparent RHTN.[46] Isolated systolic HTN (ISH) is a very common form of HTN found among older adults attributed to increased arterial stiffening. Importantly, β-AR blockers or agents that slow HR should be avoided in ISH patients because decreasing HR results in greater stroke volume (required to maintain cardiac output) and subsequent rise in SBP.[47]

NEW THERAPIES

Aprocitentan, a dual endothelin antagonist, was recently approved for use in those with RHTN by the US Food and Drug Administration (FDA) due to its efficacy in lowering office and ambulatory BP demonstrated in a prior phase-3 randomized clinical trial. In the same trial, antihypertensive effect of aprocitentan appears to be greater among older adults aged 75 or above.[48] The renal denervation (RDN) systems have recently obtained FDA approval as treatment for those with HTN. Importantly, the ultrasound RDN reduced daytime ambulatory SBP by ~4.5 mm Hg in patients with RHTN when compared with the sham-controlled study group. However, the presence of higher HR and orthostatic HTN, but not specific age groups, was associated with greater BP responses to ultrasound RDN.[49] Thus, the assessment of these pertinent factors could aid in identifying candidates for these new therapies.

Aside from these recent FDA-approved therapies, there are several others undergoing investigation for the treatment of RHTN.[50] Namely, baxdrostat and lorundrostat (aldosterone synthase inhibitors) have been shown to lower BP in adults with uncontrolled HTN. While zilebesiran, a small interfering RNA that targets and suppresses hepatic angiotensinogen production, was shown to produce a reduction in BP that lasted up to 6 months after just a single subcutaneous injection.[51]

SUMMARY

Evidence suggests that intensive BP control is both safe and effective in reducing cardiovascular events in older adults. However, because RHTN is a multifactorial disorder, a comprehensive evaluation of potential secondary causes is crucial for optimal BP control. Indeed, the successful treatment of RHTN in older adults requires proper awareness and identification of these secondary causes. Moreover, a combination of pharmacologic and nonpharmacologic interventions, such as optimal drug regimens and sodium restriction, is crucial for enhanced HTN management. As such, a shared decision-making approach with the patient, specialized care providers, and family members is necessary to promote and achieve better BP control.

CLINICS CARE POINTS

- RHTN is highly prevalent in older adults of age ≥ 60 years.
- The most common factor that can contribute to higher BP in RHTN is medication nonadherence.
- Methods to enhance medication adherence in older adults include focusing on more simplified regimens and involving family members in the treatment plan.
- Mainstay lifestyle modifications center on decreasing dietary sodium intake and increasing physical activity.
- Ensure patients are on the optimal 3-drug regimen titrated to maximally tolerated doses.
- Investigate for secondary causes of RHTN as clinically indicated.
- Utilize a shared decision-making approach with the patient to promote and achieve better BP control.

DISCLOSURE

The authors have nothing to disclose.

REFERENCES

1. Whelton PK, Carey RM, Aronow WS, et al. 2017 ACC/AHA/AAPA/ABC/ACPM/AGS/APhA/ASH/ASPC/NMA/PCNA guideline for the prevention, detection, evaluation, and management of high blood pressure in adults: executive summary: a report of the American College of Cardiology/American Heart Association Task Force on Clinical Practice Guidelines. Hypertension 2018;71:1269–324.
2. Carey RM, Calhoun DA, Bakris GL, et al. Resistant hypertension: detection, evaluation, and management: a scientific statement from the American Heart Association. Hypertension 2018;72:e53–90.
3. Chia R, Pandey A, Vongpatanasin W. Resistant hypertension-defining the scope of the problem. Prog Cardiovasc Dis 2020;63:46–50.
4. Carey RM, Sakhuja S, Calhoun DA, et al. Prevalence of apparent treatment-resistant hypertension in the United States. Hypertension 2019;73:424–31.
5. Jafari E, Cooper-DeHoff RM, Effron MB, et al. Characteristics and predictors of apparent treatment resistant hypertension in real-world populations using electronic health record-based data. Am J Hypertens 2023. https://doi.org/10.1093/ajh/hpad084.
6. de la Sierra A, Segura J, Banegas JR, et al. Clinical features of 8295 patients with resistant hypertension classified on the basis of ambulatory blood pressure monitoring. Hypertension 2011;57:898–902.
7. Tanner RM, Shimbo D, Seals SR, et al. White-coat effect among older adults: data from the Jackson Heart Study. J Clin Hypertens (Greenwich) 2016;18:139–45.
8. Melville S, Byrd JB. Out-of-Office blood pressure monitoring in 2018. JAMA 2018;320:1805–6.
9. Parodi R, Brandani L, Romero C, et al. Resistant hypertension: diagnosis, evaluation, and treatment practical approach. Eur J Intern Med 2024. https://doi.org/10.1016/j.ejim.2023.12.026.
10. Pandey A, Raza F, Velasco A, et al. Comparison of Morisky Medication Adherence Scale with therapeutic drug monitoring in apparent treatment-resistant hypertension. J Am Soc Hypertens 2015;9:420–426 e422.

11. Brinker S, Pandey A, Ayers C, et al. Therapeutic drug monitoring facilitates blood pressure control in resistant hypertension. J Am Coll Cardiol 2014;63:834–5.

12. Vitarello JA, Fitzgerald CJ, Cluett JL, et al. Prevalence of medications that may raise blood pressure among adults with hypertension in the United States. JAMA Intern Med 2022;182:90–3.

13. Qato DM, Wilder J, Schumm LP, et al. Changes in prescription and over-the-counter medication and dietary supplement use among older adults in the United States, 2005 vs 2011. JAMA Intern Med 2016;176:473–82.

14. Vaidya A, Hundemer GL, Nanba K, et al. Primary aldosteronism: state-of-the-art review. Am J Hypertens 2022;35:967–88.

15. Dluhy RG. Uncommon forms of secondary hypertension in older patients. Am J Hypertens 1998;11:52s–6s.

16. Nanba K, Vaidya A, Williams GH, et al. Age-related autonomous aldosteronism. Circulation 2017;136:347–55.

17. Burrello J, Monticone S, Losano I, et al. Prevalence of hypokalemia and primary aldosteronism in 5100 patients referred to a tertiary hypertension unit. Hypertension 2020;75:1025–33.

18. Funder JW, Carey RM, Mantero F, et al. The management of primary aldosteronism: case detection, diagnosis, and treatment: an endocrine society clinical practice guideline. J Clin Endocrinol Metab 2016;101:1889–916.

19. Patel D, Phay JE, Yen TWF, et al. Update on pheochromocytoma and paraganglioma from the sso endocrine/head and neck disease-site work group. part 1 of 2: advances in pathogenesis and diagnosis of pheochromocytoma and paraganglioma. Ann Surg Oncol 2020;27:1329–37.

20. Taieb D, Wanna GB, Ahmad M, et al. Clinical consensus guideline on the management of phaeochromocytoma and paraganglioma in patients harbouring germline SDHD pathogenic variants. Lancet Diabetes Endocrinol 2023;11:345–61.

21. Qiao N, Swearingen B, Tritos NA. Cushing's disease in older patients: presentation and outcome. Clin Endocrinol 2018;89:444–53.

22. Fleseriu M, Auchus R, Bancos I, et al. Consensus on diagnosis and management of Cushing's disease: a guideline update. Lancet Diabetes Endocrinol 2021;9: 847–75.

23. Yeghiazarians Y, Jneid H, Tietjens JR, et al. Obstructive sleep apnea and cardiovascular disease: a scientific statement from the American Heart Association. Circulation 2021;144:e56–67.

24. Thiolliere D, Harbaoui B, Falandry C, et al. Screening for hypertension-mediated organ damage and aetiology: still of value after 65 years of age? J Geriatr Cardiol 2022;19:791–801.

25. Delgado C, Baweja M, Crews DC, et al. A unifying approach for GFR Estimation: recommendations of the NKF-ASN task force on reassessing the inclusion of race in diagnosing kidney disease. Am J Kidney Dis 2022;79:268–288 e261.

26. Fu EL, Carrero JJ, Sang Y, et al. Association of low glomerular filtration rate with adverse outcomes at older age in a large population with routinely measured cystatin C. Ann Intern Med 2024. https://doi.org/10.7326/M23-1138.

27. Caps MT, Perissinotto C, Zierler RE, et al. Prospective study of atherosclerotic disease progression in the renal artery. Circulation 1998;98:2866–72.

28. Pimenta E, Gaddam KK, Oparil S, et al. Effects of dietary sodium reduction on blood pressure in subjects with resistant hypertension: results from a randomized trial. Hypertension 2009;54:475–81.

29. Hornstrup BG, Hoffmann-Petersen N, Lauridsen TG, et al. Dietary sodium restriction reduces blood pressure in patients with treatment resistant hypertension. BMC Nephrol 2023;24:274.

30. Lopes S, Mesquita-Bastos J, Garcia C, et al. Effect of exercise training on ambulatory blood pressure among patients with resistant hypertension: a randomized clinical trial. JAMA Cardiol 2021;6:1317–23.

31. Henkin JS, Pinto RS, Machado CLF, et al. Chronic effect of resistance training on blood pressure in older adults with prehypertension and hypertension: a systematic review and meta-analysis. Exp Gerontol 2023;177:112193.

32. Parthasarathy HK, Menard J, White WB, et al. A double-blind, randomized study comparing the antihypertensive effect of eplerenone and spironolactone in patients with hypertension and evidence of primary aldosteronism. J Hypertens 2011;29:980–90.

33. Baudrand R, Guarda FJ, Torrey J, et al. Dietary sodium restriction increases the risk of misinterpreting mild cases of primary aldosteronism. J Clin Endocrinol Metab 2016;101:3989–96.

34. O'Malley KJ, Alnablsi MW, Xi Y, et al. Diagnostic performance of the adrenal vein to inferior vena cava aldosterone ratio in classifying the subtype of primary aldosteronism. Hypertens Res 2023. https://doi.org/10.1038/s41440-023-01421-9.

35. Lenders JW, Duh QY, Eisenhofer G, et al. Endocrine S. Pheochromocytoma and paraganglioma: an endocrine society clinical practice guideline. J Clin Endocrinol Metab 2014;99:1915–42.

36. Nieman LK, Biller BM, Findling JW, et al. Treatment of cushing's syndrome: an endocrine society clinical practice guideline. J Clin Endocrinol Metab 2015; 100:2807–31.

37. Labarca G, Schmidt A, Dreyse J, et al. Efficacy of continuous positive airway pressure (CPAP) in patients with obstructive sleep apnea (OSA) and resistant hypertension (RH): systematic review and meta-analysis. Sleep Med Rev 2021;58: 101446.

38. Dedhia RC, Bliwise DL, Quyyumi AA, et al. Hypoglossal nerve stimulation and cardiovascular outcomes for patients with obstructive sleep apnea: a randomized clinical trial. JAMA Otolaryngol Head Neck Surg 2024;150:39–48.

39. Schwartz AR, Jacobowitz O, Eisele DW, et al. Targeted hypoglossal nerve stimulation for patients with obstructive sleep apnea: a randomized clinical trial. JAMA Otolaryngol Head Neck Surg 2023;149:512–20.

40. Murphy TP, Cooper CJ, Pencina KM, et al. Relationship of albuminuria and renal artery stent outcomes: results from the CORAL randomized clinical trial (cardiovascular outcomes with renal artery lesions). Hypertension 2016;68:1145–52.

41. Bhalla V, Textor SC, Beckman JA, et al. Revascularization for renovascular disease: a scientific statement from the American Heart Association. Hypertension 2022;79:e128–43.

42. Agarwal R, Sinha AD, Tu W. Chlorthalidone for resistant hypertension in advanced chronic kidney disease. Circulation 2022;146:718–20.

43. Williams B, MacDonald TM, Morant S, et al. Spironolactone versus placebo, bisoprolol, and doxazosin to determine the optimal treatment for drug-resistant hypertension (PATHWAY-2): a randomised, double-blind, crossover trial. Lancet 2015; 386:2059–68.

44. Williams B, MacDonald TM, Morant SV, et al. Endocrine and haemodynamic changes in resistant hypertension, and blood pressure responses to spironolactone or amiloride: the PATHWAY-2 mechanisms substudies. Lancet Diabetes Endocrinol 2018;6:464–75.

45. Kario K, Ferdinand KC, Vongpatanasin W. Are SGLT2 inhibitors new hypertension drugs? Circulation 2021;143:1750–3.

46. Jackson AM, Jhund PS, Anand IS, et al. Sacubitril-valsartan as a treatment for apparent resistant hypertension in patients with heart failure and preserved ejection fraction. Eur Heart J 2021;42:3741–52.

47. Bavishi C, Goel S, Messerli FH. Isolated systolic hypertension: an update after SPRINT. Am J Med 2016;129:1251–8.

48. Schlaich MP, Bellet M, Weber MA, et al. Dual endothelin antagonist aprocitentan for resistant hypertension (PRECISION): a multicentre, blinded, randomised, parallel-group, phase 3 trial. Lancet 2022;400:1927–37.

49. Kirtane AJ, Sharp ASP, Mahfoud F, et al. Patient-level pooled analysis of ultrasound renal denervation in the Sham-Controlled RADIANCE II, RADIANCE-HTN SOLO, and RADIANCE-HTN TRIO Trials. JAMA Cardiol 2023;8:464–73.

50. Blazek O, Bakris GL. Novel therapies on the horizon of hypertension management. Am J Hypertens 2023;36:73–81.

51. Desai AS, Webb DJ, Taubel J, et al. Zilebesiran, an RNA interference therapeutic agent for hypertension. N Engl J Med 2023;389:228–38.

Deprescribing Hypertension Medication in Older Adults
Can It Lower Drug Burden Without Causing Harm?

Marcio Galvão Oliveira, BPharm, PhD[a,b,*],
Pablo Maciel Moreira, BPharm, MsC[b,c,1],
Welma Wildes Amorim, MD, PhD[d], Kenneth Boockvar, MD, MS[e]

KEYWORDS

• Hypertension • Deprescribing • Older people • Polypharmacy

KEY POINTS

- Antihypertensives are one of the groups of medications most used by older populations, and more intensive treatment goals may have potential for adverse events.
- When planned and patient-centered, antihypertensive deprescribing has not been associated with any significant adverse outcomes.
- Antihypertensives might benefit patients with comorbidities, and they may be prescribed with a specific focus on addressing these additional health concerns. Discontinuing such agents could exacerbate the underlying conditions for which they were initially prescribed.
- A medication review considering the prescription of inappropriate antihypertensives and their gradual withdrawal should be carried out.

INTRODUCTION

Drugs are the most commonly used medical technology to treat chronic diseases, and older patients often need to use multiple drugs due to multimorbidity.[1] The drug

[a] Multidisciplinary Institute in Health, Federal University of Bahia, Brazil; [b] Postgraduate Program in Pharmaceutical Services and Policies, Federal University of Bahia, Brazil; [c] Municipal Health Department of Vitória da Conquista, Vitória da Conquista, Bahia, Brazil; [d] State University of Southwest Bahia, Department of Health Sciences, Brazil. Estrada do Bem Querer, km 4. Bairro Universitário, CEP.: 45083 -900. Vitória da Conquista – BA, Brazil; [e] Division of Gerontology, Geriatrics, and Palliative Care, University of Alabama, 933 19th Street South, Birmingham, AL 35233, USA
[1] Present address: Rua Hormindo Barros, 58 - Quadra 17, Lote 58 | CEP: 45.029-094 - Candeias, Vitória da Conquista, Bahia, Brazil.
* Corresponding author. Rua Hormindo Barros, 58 - Quadra 17, Lote 58 | CEP: 45.029-094 - Candeias, Vitória da Conquista, Bahia, Brazil.
E-mail address: mgalvao@ufba.br

Clin Geriatr Med 40 (2024) 659–668
https://doi.org/10.1016/j.cger.2024.04.012
0749-0690/24/© 2024 Elsevier Inc. All rights reserved.

geriatric.theclinics.com

burden may increase hospitalization, cognitive impairment, falls, and increased mortality in this population.[1,2] The presence of multiple health conditions, leading to the use of multiple medications (polypharmacy), along with geriatric syndromes like cognitive decline and socio-economic challenges such as loneliness or lack of informal assistance, significantly affects the quality of life for older individuals and the standard of health care they receive.[3] The challenge is making decisions based not solely on age but on carefully considering the patient's overall medical, physical, social, and mental characteristics.[3,4] Personalized medicine plays a crucial role in addressing these challenges, and health professionals must adapt their current practices to account for changes in pharmacokinetics and pharmacodynamics associated with aging.[4,5] Additionally, they should be mindful of factors such as cognitive impairment, concurrent health issues, polypharmacy, orthostatic hypotension, falls, medication cost, side effects, visual and auditory limitations, social support, caregiver availability, and frailty.[4]

Hypertension is one of the most prevalent comorbid conditions in older people, rarely occurring in isolation.[6] It is a severe disease that significantly increases the risk of heart, brain, kidney, and other diseases. Approximately 1.4 billion people globally have high blood pressure.[7] Several studies, traditionally excluding older adults, especially those aged 80 years and above, have historically concentrated on guiding the screening and management of hypertension. Although the SPRINT trial demonstrated a systolic blood pressure (SBP) of less than 120 mm Hg, as compared with less than 140 mm Hg, resulted in lower rates of fatal and nonfatal major cardiovascular events and death from any cause in individuals aged greater than 50 year without diabetes and a previous stroke,[8] the treatment of elevated blood pressure in older people remains controversial.[4,9–11] The optimal SBP targets for older patients continue to be a subject of considerable debate, as various guidelines propose different thresholds ranging from strict (<120 mm Hg) to more lenient (SBP < 140 or < 150 mm Hg based on cardiovascular risk[11]; for additional discussion, refer to Supiano[12]).

Older patients are at a higher risk of adverse reactions to hypertension overtreatment, such as postural hypotension and falls.[9] Effective pharmacologic lowering of diastolic blood pressure can potentially diminish coronary perfusion and elevate the risk of myocardial infarction. However, concerns regarding the effect of low diastolic BP have been largely dismissed.[13] The use of alpha-blockers is linked to a higher risk of heart failure. Older individuals who persist in taking blood pressure medications despite experiencing hypotension face elevated risks of mortality and hospital admissions.[10] Moreover, the utilization of antihypertensive drugs is linked to adverse effects such as orthostatic hypotension, metabolic impacts, frailty, dizziness, syncope, falls, and, in certain studies, a potential deterioration in cognitive function among individuals with dementia.[14]

Mitigating harm associated with medication is especially challenging within the framework of multimorbidity and polypharmacy. However, judicious management of multiple medications may be warranted and advantageous in addressing intricate comorbidities in older patients, mainly when each drug is thoughtfully evaluated in the context of the patient's overall health and prognosis.[15] Polypharmacy is the concurrent use of multiple medications and is often defined as the routine use of 5 or more drugs. This includes over-the-counter prescription and traditional and complementary medicines a patient uses. The objective should be to minimize unwarranted polypharmacy, characterized by the imprudent prescription of an excessive number of medications, and promote justified polypharmacy. This involves the rational prescription of multiple drugs founded on the best available evidence while considering individual patient factors and the specific context of their health.[16]

The global prevalence of polypharmacy is on the rise, particularly among older adults, and mainly encompasses prescription drugs. The number of daily medications tends to be generally proportional to the concurrent presence of chronic medical conditions.[15] Deprescribing is the process of withdrawal of an inappropriate medication, supervised by a health care professional to manage polypharmacy and improve outcomes.[17] Knowledge of potential adverse effects and consideration of patient factors across physical, social, and psychological domains is essential for deprescribing.[18]

WHO CAN BENEFIT FROM ANTIHYPERTENSIVE DEPRESCRIBING?

One component of good prescribing is deprescribing[19,20]; however, clinical guidelines frequently focus on how and when an antihypertensive medication should be initiated. There is often no information about when and how such drugs should be deprescribed, with clinical trials foregoing the opportunity to collect data on the effects of stopping antihypertensive medication during or at the end of the study period.[11] A strategy of deprescribing proves valuable when the ongoing antihypertensive regimen no longer corresponds to the care objectives, especially in scenarios like end-of-life care, where the potential for additional cardiovascular disease (CVD) or other prevention benefits is negligible. In these instances, deprescribing may be considered an acknowledgment of therapeutic futility. Also, antihypertensive medications might become unsuitable for individuals at a heightened risk of adverse events (**Table 1**).[21,22]

An essential aspect of deprescribing involves identifying medications that may be inappropriate for withdrawal in high-risk patients, aiming to prevent potential adverse events. However, this task is complex, as determining who is at high risk poses challenges. Moreover, this approach is not without risks itself, as discontinuing an antihypertensive medication to prevent a fall might inadvertently increase the likelihood of a more severe cardiovascular event, such as a stroke.[22] In response to this challenge, tools and guidelines have been developed to assist clinicians in evaluating the appropriateness of medications, facilitating the deprescribing of potentially inappropriate medications (PIMs), and recommending suitable alternatives, particularly for vulnerable populations.[23,24] These resources can support the entire deprescribing process or focus on specific aspects.[24] They may take an explicit approach, offering predefined criteria or lists of medications, or an implicit approach, relying on clinical judgment and expert opinion.

Some tools combine explicit and implicit methods to assess the appropriateness of medications.[23,24] Considering cultural, societal, and medical diversity, various tools and guidelines have been created to accommodate multiple health care settings. These resources aim to empower clinicians, aiding them in decision-making and enhancing their self-efficacy in medication management to improve care for vulnerable groups.[23] The 2 main sources of information about PIMs for older adults are the American Geriatrics Society Beers Criteria and STOPP/START.[25,26]

Older individuals are notably susceptible to the white coat effect, a clinical phenomenon wherein the systolic and diastolic blood pressure measured in a clinical setting is higher than the readings obtained through home blood pressure monitoring.[9,27] This transient change in blood pressure substantially impacts signs and symptoms and may lead to overtreatment, leading to errors in decision-making, thereby complicating treatment.[9] Almost 20% of hypertensive patients may have a white coat effect detected through blood pressure measurement at home, compared to the office measurement. The mean difference in blood pressure between the places can reach 10.1 mm Hg for systolic and 4.3 mm Hg for diastolic.[27] Relying solely on a single office blood pressure measurement may result in unnecessary treatment with antihypertensive drugs,

Table 1
Discontinuing antihypertensive medication criteria and rationale for deprescribing in older people

Discontinuing Antihypertensive Medication Criteria	Rationale
White coat effect	For patients whose office blood pressure is above target when taking medication, it is suggested to check blood pressure at home.[30] If blood pressure is at goal on home blood pressure monitoring, or the patient has symptoms of hypotension, deprescribing antihypertensive medication should be considered.[9]
Orthostatic hypotension	Asymptomatic orthostatic hypotension is prevalent in older people. Excessive prescribing of antihypertensive medications targeting seated systolic blood pressure readings may occur in more than one-fourth of geriatric patients.[29]
Potentially inappropriate prescription	Potentially inappropriate medications, which have low evidence of effectiveness and a high risk of adverse events, should be deprescribed in older people, for example, central alpha-agonists and non-selective peripheral alpha-1 blockers for the treatment of hypertension.[26]
High-risk patients	Several older patients are at high risk of adverse reactions to antihypertensive treatment and this risk outweighs the benefits of treatment. In some cases, it may be inappropriate to deprescribe antihypertensive medications, especially if they have been prescribed for indications other than blood pressure management.[30] Deprescribing should occur when adverse drug events occur (eg, electrolyte disorders, falling from low blood pressure), when the regimen appears to be "overaggressive" (eg, blood pressure <110), or when blood pressure control is not consistent with goals of care (eg, end of life)
Prescribing cascades	Each antihypertensive class has predictable adverse effects that while, typically mild, may lead to predictable prescribing cascades. Drug-induced symptoms frequently go under reported and when reported are often misattributed as the manifestation of new disease.[29]

primarily due to the white coat effect. Home blood pressure monitoring is a safe and straightforward approach for identifying cases influenced by the white coat effect. This method allows for adjustments in dosage or medication, thereby mitigating unnecessary risks, particularly in the case of older patients.[9] (Additional information is provided in Burks C et al.[28])

Another essential clinical condition is orthostatic hypotension, which is prevalent in the older population[29] (between 30% and 50%)[11] and may be underdiagnosed. In an observational study, individuals aged 65 years or older, capable of standing, underwent screening for orthostatic hypotension. This condition was defined as a reduction in SBP of 20 mm Hg or greater or diastolic blood pressure of 10 mm Hg or greater after standing for 3 minutes. Clinic personnel measured sitting blood pressure after patients had been quietly seated in the examination room. Subsequently, patients stood for approximately 3 minutes, and blood pressure was recorded while standing. The prevalence of orthostatic hypotension was 18%. Physicians were more inclined to discontinue antihypertensive medication in patients who screened positive for orthostatic hypotension compared to those who did not.[29]

High-risk patients are individuals whose characteristics and medical history predispose them to an elevated risk of adverse events associated with antihypertensive therapy. These risk factors encompass advancing age, dementia, chronic kidney disease, prior adverse drug reactions, blood pressure maintained below 110 to 120 mm Hg (indicating overaggressive antihypertensive treatment), polypharmacy, and frailty. Adverse drug reactions may manifest as hypotension, syncope, falls, fractures, acute kidney injury, and electrolyte abnormalities. Certain antihypertensive classes may contribute to specific adverse reactions, such as acute kidney injury and electrolyte imbalances, while others are more closely associated with lowering blood pressure (eg, hypotension and syncope). Numerous conditions and factors may contribute to an individual's heightened risk of experiencing adverse events.[30]

Another effective strategy within deprescribing initiatives involves identifying prevalent prescribing cascades, where a second (potentially preventable) medication is prescribed in response to an adverse effect or drug reaction induced by another medication. For instance, the initiation of calcium channel blockers, known for causing peripheral edema, may lead clinicians to prescribe diuretics to mitigate this adverse effect. Another example is the common practice of prescribing antihypertensives following the initiation of nonsteroidal anti-inflammatories. Additionally, numerous widely used medications, including corticosteroids, estrogens, testosterones, certain antidepressants, and common over-the-counter cold remedies and supplements, may contribute to elevated blood pressure levels.[31,32]

WHAT ARE THE BENEFITS OR HARMS?

The ECSTATIC study examined the effect of deprescribing cardiovascular medications in community-dwelling patients aged 40 to 70 years. In this cluster, randomized nonblinded parallel-group active-control noninferiority study, general practitioners and practitioner nurses were trained to follow deprescribing guidelines for gradual dose reduction and monitoring blood pressure and cholesterol levels. No intervention was planned for the usual care group. The findings indicated that attempting to discontinue preventive cardiovascular medication in general practice patients with a predicted low 10 year CVD risk was deemed safe in the short term compared to standard care, with only a minimal difference observed in the increase of predicted 10 year CVD risk. However, after 2 years, 65% of the 1067 participants stopped a statin or antihypertensive, and 27% could maintain this. Compared to the usual care group, SBP was 6 mm Hg higher for the intervention group, and diastolic blood pressure was 4 mm Hg higher. Cost and quality-adjusted life years did not differ between the groups.[33]

In 2020, a Cochrane Review evaluated 6 trials involving 1073 participants aged 50 years and older, focusing on deprescribing antihypertensive medications for indications such as hypertension and/or primary prevention of CVD. The duration and follow-up of these trials varied from 3 to 12 months, and this short term was a limitation of these studies. The analysis revealed no significant impact on the primary endpoints of all-cause mortality (odds ratio [OR] 2.08, 95% confidence interval [CI] 0.79–5.46) or myocardial infarction (OR 1.86, 95% CI 0.19–17.98) when comparing the discontinuation and continuation of antihypertensives. Additionally, antihypertensive deprescribing did not show to increase the risk of adverse events.[34]

The OPTIMISE trial investigated deprescribing of a single antihypertensive medication in participants aged 80 years or older, with a baseline SBP of less than 150 mm Hg (mean baseline 130 mm Hg) and already under treatment with 2 or more antihypertensives. Participants were randomized to a strategy of antihypertensive medication reduction (removal of 1 drug) or usual care, in which no medication changes were mandated. Primary care physicians participating in the study were provided with a medication reduction algorithm. They evaluated the medication regimens of each patient before the baseline. They determined which antihypertensive drug would be discontinued if the participant was assigned to the medication reduction group of the trial. Compared to the standard care group, most participants achieved the primary endpoint, maintaining an SBP less than 150 mm Hg at the 12 week follow-up (87.7% vs 86.4%, relative risk [RR] 0.98, 95% CI 0.92–1.05). Following the reduction in medication, the mean increase in SBP was 3.4 mm Hg (95% CI, 1.1–5.8 mm Hg). There were no significant differences in serious adverse effects. Two-thirds of the intervention group did not require any adjustments to their regimen after discontinuing the antihypertensive, indicating that successful withdrawal may be attainable for many patients.[35]

A limitation of these studies is the short duration in assessing the long-term impact and potential harm associated with antihypertensive medication withdrawal. The low harm observed during these trials does not definitively exclude the possibility of adverse events occurring over a more extended period. The delayed onset of complications, such as cardiovascular events, underscores the need for extended follow-up to comprehensively evaluate the safety profile of deprescribing interventions.

HOW TO DEPRESCRIBE ANTIHYPERTENSIVE DRUGS?

Although evidence supports the effectiveness and pharmacoeconomic benefits of deprescribing interventions, there is considerable heterogeneity in the types of interventions and the reporting of processes.[36]

Effective clinical practice should incorporate shared decision-making, wherein health care professionals discuss the risks and benefits of various treatment options with patients and their caregivers. However, it is recognized that implementing shared decision-making can pose challenges in the practical application of deprescribing.[37]

The initial step in determining the appropriateness of antihypertensive deprescribing involves obtaining accurate blood pressure measurements, particularly in older patients.[9] Accurately and consistently measuring blood pressure multiple times is essential for establishing a comprehensive profile of blood pressure peaks and troughs. This profile is crucial for making well-informed decisions regarding antihypertensives and setting blood pressure targets. In the older population, blood pressure readings demonstrate more significant variability than in the general population, and even slight variations in blood pressure measurement techniques can lead to significant effects. To ensure precision, blood pressure measurements should consider factors such as appropriate cuff size, simultaneous measurement on both arms (except in cases of unilateral subclavian artery stenosis), adjustments for underlying atrial fibrillation where cardiac stroke volume and blood pressure may vary beat by beat, and measurements taken in both lying and standing positions.[11] After measuring blood pressure in the sitting position, repeat the measurement in the standing position after 3 minutes and assess the possibility of orthostatic hypotension.[29] Home or ambulatory blood pressure measurements should be performed whenever possible.[9]

It is essential to conduct a thorough review of the medications taken by patients and engage in discussion with them regarding the outcomes and care goals. Patients should be informed about the evidence supporting the benefits of drugs that may be questionable. Collaborating with pharmacists and other health care professionals, engaging in discussions with patients and their caregivers, and utilizing clinical tools are valuable approaches that can assist physicians in optimizing medication lists and undertaking appropriate deprescribing when necessary.[38]

Tools such as STOPP/START[24] and the American Geriatrics Society Beers' criteria[26] can identify potentially inappropriate antihypertensive medications. Discontinuing antihypertensive medications may not be advisable, mainly if they were prescribed for reasons other than managing blood pressure. Antihypertensive medications should be tapered off sequentially, one at a time, with a 4 week interval between each withdrawal. When discontinuing beta-blockers, diuretics, or any other antihypertensive drugs prescribed at high doses, health care professionals should initially contemplate dose reduction before complete cessation. It is crucial to monitor the patient's SBP 4 weeks after discontinuing therapy to ensure it remains within the target range. In cases of uncontrolled blood pressure, health care professionals should contemplate reintroducing the previously discontinued medication at a lower dose (if feasible) or suggest alternative non-pharmacological strategies to effectively manage blood pressure.[22]

Additionally, it may be crucial to consider both blood pressure levels and cardiovascular risk, as continued treatment may remain suitable and beneficial for certain patients with multiple risk factors.[30] Agents with antihypertensive effects may benefit patients with other comorbidities and may be prescribed more specifically for these additional purposes.[11] Discontinuing beta-blockers for heart failure, atrial fibrillation, or ischemic heart disease, angiotensin converting-enzyme (ACE) inhibitors for heart failure or renal protection, and prazosin for prostatic symptoms could exacerbate the underlying medical conditions.[30]

CLINICS CARE POINTS

- Deprescribing antihypertensives in older adults should consider the active participation of patients and caregivers.
- Blood pressure measurements must be accurate: the effect of the white coat and orthostatic hypotension must be evaluated.
- A medication review considering the prescription of inappropriate antihypertensives and their gradual withdrawal should be carried out.
- Patients should be monitored continuously, and cardiovascular risk should be assessed.

DISCLOSURE

The authors have nothing to disclose.

FUNDING

This study was financed in part by the Coordenação de Aperfeiçoamento de Pessoal de Nível Superior – Brasil (CAPES) – Finance Code 001, US Deprescribing Research Network and the National Institute on Aging (Grant number R24AG064025).

REFERENCES

1. Wang Y, Li X, Jia D, et al. Exploring polypharmacy burden among elderly patients with chronic diseases in Chinese community: a cross-sectional study. BMC Geriatr 2021;21(1):308. https://doi.org/10.1186/s12877-021-02247-1.

2. Masnoon N, Shakib S, Kalisch-Ellett L, et al. What is polypharmacy? A systematic review of definitions. BMC Geriatr 2017;17(1):230. https://doi.org/10.1186/s12877-017-0621-2.

3. Roller-Wirnsberger R, Thurner B, Pucher C, et al. The clinical and therapeutic challenge of treating older patients in clinical practice. Br J Clin Pharmacol 2020;86(10):1904–11.

4. Oliveros E, Patel H, Kyung S, et al. Hypertension in older adults: Assessment, management, and challenges. Clin Cardiol 2020;43(2):99–107.

5. Mangoni AA, Jackson SH. Age-related changes in pharmacokinetics and pharmacodynamics: basic principles and practical applications. Br J Clin Pharmacol 2004;57(1):6–14.

6. Chowdhury SR, Chandra Das D, Sunna TC, et al. Global and regional prevalence of multimorbidity in the adult population in community settings: a systematic review and meta-analysis. eClinicalMedicine 2023;57. https://doi.org/10.1016/j.eclinm.2023.101860.

7. World Health Organization. Guideline for the pharmacological treatment of hypertension in adults. Geneva: WHO; 2021.

8. Wright JT Jr, Williamson JD, Whelton PK, et al. A randomized trial of intensive versus standard blood-pressure control. N Engl J Med 2015;373(22):2103–16.

9. Moreira PM, Aguiar EC, Castro PR, et al. Optimizing hypertension treatment in older patients through home blood pressure monitoring by pharmacists in primary care: the MINOR clinical trial. Clin Ther 2023. https://doi.org/10.1016/j.clinthera.2023.06.007.

10. Shantsila E, Lip GYH, Shantsila A, et al. Antihypertensive treatment in people of very old age with frailty: time for a paradigm shift? J Hypertens 2023;41(10):1502–10.

11. Scott IA, Hilmer SN, Le Couteur DG. Going beyond the guidelines in Individualising the Use of antihypertensive drugs in older patients. Drugs Aging 2019;36(8):675–85.

12. Supiano M.A., Optimal Blood Pressure Targets with Age. Clin Geriatr Med, 40 (4), 2024, [Epub ahead of print].

13. Beddhu S, Chertow GM, Cheung AK, et al. Influence of baseline diastolic blood pressure on effects of intensive compared with standard blood pressure control. Circulation 2018;137(2):134–43.

14. Raghunandan R, Howard K, Ilomaki J, et al. Preferences for deprescribing antihypertensive medications amongst clinicians, carers and people living with dementia: a discrete choice experiment. Age Ageing 2023;52(8). https://doi.org/10.1093/ageing/afad153.

15. Daunt R, Curtin D, O'Mahony D. Polypharmacy stewardship: a novel approach to tackle a major public health crisis. The Lancet Healthy Longevity 2023;4(5):e228–35.

16. Health World. Organization.Medication safety in polypharmacy: technical report. Geneva: WHO; 2019.

17. Reeve E, Gnjidic D, Long J, et al. A systematic review of the emerging definition of 'deprescribing' with network analysis: implications for future research and clinical practice. Br J Clin Pharmacol 2015;80(6):1254–68.

18. Aggarwal P, Woolford SJ, Patel HP. Multi-morbidity and polypharmacy in older people: challenges and Opportunities for clinical practice. Geriatrics 2020;5(4):85.

19. Farrell B, Mangin D. Deprescribing is an essential Part of good prescribing. Am Fam Physician 2019;99(1):7–9.

20. Amorim WW, Passos LC, Oliveira MG. Why deprescribing instead of not prescribing? Geriatrics, Gerontology and Aging 2020;14(4):294–7.

21. Jowett S, Kodabuckus S, Ford GA, et al. Cost-effectiveness of antihypertensive deprescribing in primary care: a Markov Modelling study using data from the OPTiMISE trial. Hypertension 2022;79(5):1122–31.

22. Sheppard JP, Benetos A, McManus RJ. Antihypertensive deprescribing in older adults: a practical guide. Curr Hypertens Rep 2022;24(11):571–80.

23. Anlay DZ, Paque K, Van Leeuwen E, et al. Tools and guidelines to assess the appropriateness of medication and aid deprescribing: an umbrella review. Br J Clin Pharmacol 2024;90(1):12–106.

24. Oliveira MG, Amorim WW, de Jesus SR, et al. A comparison of the Beers and STOPP criteria for identifying the use of potentially inappropriate medications among elderly patients in primary care. J Eval Clin Pract 2015;21(2):320–5.

25. O'Mahony D, Cherubini A, Guiteras AR, et al. STOPP/START criteria for potentially inappropriate prescribing in older people: version 3. European Geriatric Medicine 2023;1–8.

26. American Geriatrics Society. 2023 updated AGS Beers Criteria® for potentially inappropriate medication use in older adults. J Am Geriatr Soc 2023;71(7): 2052–81.

27. Moreno JN, Amorim WW, Mistro S, et al. Evaluation of blood pressure through home monitoring in brazilian primary care: a feasibility study. Ciência Saúde Coletiva 2021;26(8):2997–3004.

28. Burks C, Shimbo D, Bowling CB. Long-term monitoring of blood pressure in older adults: a focus on self-measured blood pressure monitoring. Clin Geriatr Med, 40 (4), 2024, [Epub ahead of print].

29. Kaye MG, Rutowski J, Aftab H, et al. Screening for orthostatic hypotension in the geriatric population in a real-world primary care setting reduces prescribed antihypertensive medications. Blood Press Monit 2023;28(6):338–42.

30. Sheppard JP, Benetos A, Bogaerts J, et al. Strategies for identifying patients for deprescribing of blood pressure medications in routine practice: an evidence review. Curr Hypertens Rep 2024. https://doi.org/10.1007/s11906-024-01293-5.

31. Anderson TS, Steinman MA. Antihypertensive prescribing cascades as high-Priority targets for deprescribing. JAMA Intern Med 2020;180(5):651–2.

32. Weinfeld JM, Hart KM, Vargas JD. Home blood pressure monitoring. Am Fam Physician 2021;104(3):237–43.

33. Luymes CH, Poortvliet RKE, van Geloven N, et al. Deprescribing preventive cardiovascular medication in patients with predicted low cardiovascular disease risk in general practice – the ECSTATIC study: a cluster randomised non-inferiority trial. BMC Med 2018;16(1):5.

34. Reeve E, Jordan V, Thompson W, et al. Withdrawal of antihypertensive drugs in older people. Cochrane Database Syst Rev 2020;6(6):Cd012572.

35. Sheppard JP, Burt J, Lown M, et al. Effect of antihypertensive medication reduction vs usual care on short-term blood pressure control in patients with hypertension aged 80 Years and older: the OPTIMISE randomized clinical trial. JAMA 2020;323(20):2039–51.

36. Mangin D, Lamarche L, Templeton JA, et al. Theoretical Underpinnings of a Model to Reduce polypharmacy and its Negative health effects: Introducing

the Team approach to polypharmacy evaluation and reduction (TAPER). Drugs Aging 2023;40(9):857–68.

37. Ouellet N, Bergeron A-S, Gagnon E, et al. Prescribing and deprescribing in very old age: perceptions of very old adults, caregivers and health professionals. Age Ageing 2022;51(11). https://doi.org/10.1093/ageing/afac244.

38. Frank C. Deprescribing: a new word to guide medication review. CMAJ (Can Med Assoc J) 2014;186(6):407–8.

Public Health Messaging to Older Adults About Hypertension

Jared A. Spitz, MD[a],*, Eugene Yang, MD, MS[b,c],
Roger S. Blumenthal, MD[d], Garima Sharma, MD[a,e,1]

KEYWORDS

• Hypertension • Public health messaging • Older adults

KEY POINTS

• Hypertension is a major risk factor for cardiovascular disease with its prevalence and severity increasing with age.

• Older patients often do not receive adequate treatment due to therapeutic inertia as well as concerns for frailty, susceptibility to falls, and polypharmacy.

• Individuals frequently rely on online sources of health care information as do providers for ongoing medical education and updates on clinical practice guidelines.

• Public health messaging plays an important role in raising awareness and providing education to both patients and providers about hypertension in older adults.

• Public health messaging to older adults must consider changes in cognition and sensory (hearing, speech, and vision) changes that can occur with age. They must also take into account the role of family, friends, and the community in caring for older adults.

INTRODUCTION

Hypertension is a major modifiable risk factor for cardiovascular disease.[1,2] It is a well-recognized mediator of atherosclerotic cardiovascular disease[3], heart failure,[2] atrial

[a] Inova Schar Heart and Vascular, Inova Health System, 8081 Innovation Park Drive, #700, Inova Specialty Center, Fairfax, VA 22031, USA; [b] Department of Medicine, Division of Cardiology, University of Washington School of Medicine, Seattle, WA, USA; [c] UW Medicine Cardiovascular Wellness and Prevention Program, Medicine, UW Medicine - Eastside Specialty Center, Carl and Renée Behnke Endowed Professorship for Asian Health, 3100 Northup Way Box 356005 Bellevue, WA 98004, USA; [d] Ciccarone Center for the Prevention of Cardiovascular Disease, Johns Hopkins University School of Medicine, 601 North Caroline Street, Suite 7200, Baltimore, MD 21287, USA; [e] Ciccarone Center for the Prevention of Cardiovascular Disease, Johns Hopkins University School of Medicine, Baltimore, MD, USA
[1] Present address: 8081 Innovation Park Drive 700, Fairfax, VA 22031.
* Corresponding author. 8081 Innovation Park Drive, #700, Inova Specialty Center, Fairfax, VA 22031.
E-mail address: jared.spitz@inova.org
Twitter: @Jspitz_MD (J.A.S.)

Clin Geriatr Med 40 (2024) 669–683
https://doi.org/10.1016/j.cger.2024.04.006
0749-0690/24/© 2024 Elsevier Inc. All rights reserved.

fibrillation,[4] chronic kidney disease,[5] and neurocognitive decline. The prevalence and severity of hypertension increase with age[1,3,4] and disproportionately impact our older population, which is defined by the World Health Organization as individuals ≥65 year old. By 2030, this group is projected to make up around 20% of the global population.[6] The US National Health and Nutrition Examination Survey reports that 70% of adults ≥65 year old have hypertension, with this percentage expected to increase as the population continues to age.[7]

Older patients, despite having the highest prevalence of hypertension and being at the greatest risk for cardiovascular morbidity and mortality, often do not receive adequate treatment for their blood pressure (BP). This is primarily due to concerns regarding their frailty,[8] susceptibility to falls, declining renal function, and polypharmacy,[9] leading to higher rates of therapeutic inertia.[10]

A concerted public health effort to address hypertension in older adults is crucial and timely. This effort should focus on both clinicians and patients. Older adults constitute the largest group utilizing health care services and often seek medical information from sources other than their clinicians.[11]

In today's digital age, individuals of all generations frequently rely on online sources for health care information, just as health care professionals do for ongoing medical education and updates on clinical trials and important society guidelines. This trend signifies a rapidly growing platform for public health communication. The coronavirus disease 2019 pandemic has highlighted numerous opportunities and obstacles in utilizing digital media to disseminate health-related information and encourage healthy behaviors.[12] This analysis assesses the current landscape of public messaging regarding hypertension in the elderly, focusing on (1) essential elements of public health messaging, (2) establishing a framework for customized initiatives to engage the public and health care workforce, and (3) proposing solutions to existing challenges in addressing hypertension among older adults.

THE IMPORTANCE OF STREAMLINING PUBLIC HEALTH MESSAGING

Public health messaging has the potential to effectively educate both health care professionals and the general public about health care matters and offer general medical guidance.[11] Specifically for hypertension, it is crucial to streamline management approaches and clearly explain the significance of hypertension, considering that it is mostly an asymptomatic condition.[9,13–15]

In addition to patient education, public health messaging can reduce misconceptions about hypertension management (ie, tighter control of BP will not necessarily yield the same benefit in the older population, antihypertensive therapy is poorly tolerated, and so forth) and increase the confidence in these strategies and goals of care.[14]

There has been an increasing focus by public health officials and health policy makers to create strategies that can modify beliefs and behaviors and to develop communication messaging campaigns that can change health behaviors.[13] This urgency is described in detail in Healthy People 2010, where the important role of communication on modifying behavioral risk is highlighted.[16] While current public health messages are developed using models and theories available from behavior change research,[17] there is a focus on streamlining strategies toward long-term change by constructs that incorporate recipient characteristics that may affect the respondent's barriers to behavior change. Using behavioral constructs for creating messages is challenging because they require a high degree of knowledge about the message recipient through assessment of characteristics such as attitudes, motivations, and perceived self-efficacy (ie, belief in one's ability to produce an outcome). Although these models have been useful in providing general guidance for creating health messages, they offer a broad conceptual basis rather than specific guidance in message construction[16,17] (**Fig. 1**).

A FRAMEWORK FOR ENGAGING THE PUBLIC AND HEALTH CARE WORKFORCE

1. Understanding the goals and target audience

The objective of a public health campaign on hypertension in older adults is to ultimately enhance awareness and management of the condition. A key driver of suboptimal guideline adherence is therapeutic inertia, often guided by clinician concerns about patient frailty and treatment side effects. Therapeutic inertia is defined as the failure of clinicians to initiate or intensify guideline-directed therapy.[9,18,19]

According to the American Heart Association (AHA) 2024 heart disease and stroke statistics, based on current treatment thresholds for hypertension, only about 25% of hypertensive individuals have their BP controlled to optimal levels; notably, this percentage is higher ($\sim$35%) for individuals greater than 60 year old.[18] A major contributor to poor BP control rates is therapeutic inertia.[19] One large cohort study of $\sim$7300 individuals (average age 62 years; 40% female) suggested that only 13% of visits for hypertension resulted in intensification of therapy when BP was elevated; further, there was an inverse relationship between BP control and therapeutic inertia (systolic BP decreased by an average of 7 mm Hg in those in the lowest quintile for a therapeutic inertia vs a rise in systolic BP by an average of 2 mm Hg in those with the highest quintile for a therapeutic inertia score, $P<.001$).[10,19] Additionally, older age is a significant contributor to therapeutic inertia.[19]

Differences in BP guideline treatment targets and thresholds across the globe, specifically for older patients, remain a significant challenge. The 2017 American College of Cardiology (ACC) and AHA[20] BP guidelines do not have different treatment thresholds based on age. They recommend treatment to a target systolic BP less than 130 mm Hg for adults $\geq$65 year old.[20] For older adults with significant comorbidities or limited life expectancy, clinical judgment, patient preference, and a team-based approach should

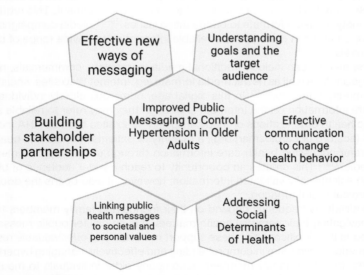

Fig. 1. A framework for public health messaging for hypertension in older adults.

be employed to determine treatment goals.[20] Conversely, 2023 European Society of Hypertension (ESH) guidelines do recommend different treatment goals based on age. For individuals 65 to 79 years old, the threshold for initiation of treatment is ≥140/90 mm Hg, with a target BP less than 140/80 mm Hg or less than 130/80 mm Hg, if tolerated. For patients greater than 80 year old, the threshold for treatment initiation is systolic BP ≥160 mm Hg with BP target of 140 to 159 mm Hg; lower initiation thresholds and targets can be considered.[21] The ESH guidelines also provide specific strategies on how to personalize BP treatment goals based on an assessment of frailty that accounts for a patient's ability to perform activities of daily living, the presence or absence of memory impairment, and overall functional status.[21] Most hypertension guidelines recommend clinical judgment, shared decision-making, and a team-based approach to determine treatment targets for older adults.[19,21,22] Clinicians must balance the cardiovascular benefits of treating hypertension in older adults against frailty and the risk of falls or orthostatic hypotension.[22–24] BP treatment targets based on frailty status can be useful in therapeutic decisions as noted in the European guidelines.[21] Therefore, care of older adults should combine evidence-based management, comprehensive geriatric assessments, and team-based coordination.[8,9,25,26]

2. Developing an effective communication strategy focusing on health behaviors

There are several key factors to address in health messaging aimed at older patients including an emphasis on regular health checkups and early detection and monitoring of BP. This is especially true given the need to balance side effects with the importance of BP treatment.[8] Encouraging patients to ask their clinicians about BP control is essential. A strong emphasis should also be placed on sustained lifestyle optimization. Many public health campaigns highlight the importance of lifestyle modifications, such as a healthy diet, regular exercise, and stress management to treat hypertension.[13,27] Measurement of BP is an essential tool for diagnosing hypertension and monitoring response to treatment. Initiatives aimed at encouraging individuals to get their BP checked and educating them on the correct way to measure their BP improve diagnosis and adherence.[28]

An effective communication strategy in older patients must address potential cognitive and sensory limitations such as visual and hearing impairment. This requires utilizing a variety of media formats to bridge these issues.[29–51] Media campaigns should be developed that can communicate reliable information to a wide range of comprehension levels.[29,30,48]

These strategies can include traditional media (pamphlets, commercials, newspapers, magazines) as well as newer media formats (eg, Internet Web sites, social media) and community outreach.[30,31] In this digital age, numerous elderly individuals seek health care information on the Internet.[32] Although they may refer to reliable sources like public health organizations or medical society Web sites such as AHA (heart.org) and ACC (acc.org or cardiosmart.org), a majority of patients with chronic health conditions prefer accessing health care information through unconventional means like social media.[31,33] This creates an opportunity to reach a wider audience of older patients with scientifically validated information; however, it also opens the door to potential medical misinformation.[33]

Older individuals frequently depend on their friends and family members to assist them in navigating their personal health matters. It is crucial for public messaging to acknowledge the significance of these support networks and offer valuable resources and information to aid them in comprehending and effectively managing hypertension. Oftentimes, friends or family members accompany older individuals to medical appointments, acting as advocates and taking notes on their behalf.[34]

Additionally, with the proliferation of online health resources, older adults frequently seek out information online. There was a 5-fold increase in Internet use by individuals older than age 65 years old between 2000 and 2016.[31] However, Internet use does not equate with comfort of use, so friends and family are often called upon to serve as guides to bridge this digital divide.[34] To this end, messaging that respects the role of friends and family is crucial.

3. Addressing social determinants of health and their association with hypertension

Social determinants of health, defined as "conditions in the environments where people are born, live, learn, work, play, worship, and age that affect a wide range of health, functioning, and quality-of-life outcomes and risks,"[35] broadly impact health care outcomes, including BP control.[35,36] Older adults often experience declines in income, social isolation and loneliness, and reduced mobility.[37] Additionally, they are more likely to have chronic illnesses that require frequent encounters with the health care system.[35] As discussed in the following sections, communication with older adults must be tailored to the specific needs of this population.

An additional factor facing in the aging population is limited or poor access to geriatric care specialists.[38,39] Although a 55% increase in the number of geriatric patients is projected by 2030, there has been a 15% to 20% decline in the number of geriatricians between 2000 and 2010[38] with an additional 10% drop forecasted between 2018 and 2030.[40]

Considering the diverse range of cardiovascular illnesses, comorbid conditions, cognitive and mental health issues, frailty, and social circumstances (eg, financial stability, social support network) that older adults may experience, it is essential to customize their care to address these factors and how those may influence their treatment.[39]

4. Linking public health messages to societal and personal values

Public messages that resonate with societal and personal values are more likely to lead to behavioral change. Within a community, tremendous value may be placed on social support networks, community leaders, and faith-based institutions.[6,34] This can range from interventions such as advising individuals to discuss their BP with clinicians to hypertension screening. In a study of Black-owned barbershops, significant BP reduction was achieved when encouragement of healthy lifestyle choices was coupled with pharmacist-led medication treatment (mean change in SBP between intervention and control group of -21.6 mm Hg (95% CI -28.4 to -14.7 mm Hg), $P < .001$); notably there was improvement in BP control even when barber-only encouragement was provided.[41]

Messaging to lay spiritual leaders to encourage discussion about hypertension can spur whole communities to engage proactively in getting screened and treated for hypertension.

In the Faith-Based Approaches in the Treatment of Hypertension trial,[42] 8 churches (n = 373) were randomized into 2 groups. In one group, lay health advisors from the church community delivered a series of group sessions focused on therapeutic lifestyle changes followed by several sessions of motivational interviewing. These sessions incorporated elements of prayer and faith-based discussions. The second group received 1 session on therapeutic lifestyle change followed by a series of lectures from local health experts; both groups received a similar number of sessions. The primary outcome of BP control at 6 months showed a statistically significant systolic BP reduction of ~ 6 mm Hg ($P = .029$; -10.99- -0.59) in the group that participated in the sessions delivered by lay health advisors.[42]

Qualitative survey data from Thailand[43] revealed that individuals who had a stronger sense of community and higher spiritual engagement were more inclined to adopt healthy behaviors to manage their BP. Individuals who were actively working to manage their BP also described feeling happier and more willing to engage with family and their social networks.[43] These studies highlight the significant impact that local communities and religious institutions can have in facilitating individuals' involvement in their health care, making them excellent candidates for public health initiatives. Additionally, as many of these institutions are linked with marginalized communities, these efforts could assist in providing access to resources for these communities to alleviate significant disparities in health care access.

5. Building stakeholder partnerships (industry, government, healthy policy)

There are a number of groups that will play a key role in developing public health messaging to older individuals about hypertension. Relevant stakeholders and their possible roles are shown in **Table 1**.[44] Additionally, technology companies play an increasingly important role in tracking health care data. Making sure that these technologies are user friendly for older patients is critical.[45] Additionally, major search engine companies should promote credible health information using search engine optimization algorithms.[30]

6. Finding patient centered strategies to improve public health messaging

It is essential to use clear and concise language in order to effectively communicate with patients.[17] This is particularly important when considering the diverse population that a public health campaign aims to reach. Therefore, it is crucial to employ culturally sensitive language and strategies. It is important to take into account health literacy, readability of materials, and potential sensory deficits like hearing and visual impairment when interacting with an older demographic.[17,46–52]

The US Center for Disease Control and Prevention *Healthy People* report defined health literacy as "the degree to which individuals have the capacity to obtain, process, and understand basic health information and services needed to make appropriate health decisions."[46] Patients older than 65 years of age demonstrate the lowest level of "proficient" health literacy (3%) and the highest level of "below basic" health literacy (29%).[46] A recent study[47] suggests that only 55% of older patients understand their BP numbers, which impacted their willingness to act on care recommendations.

In addition to health literacy, written communication must be both understandable and reliable.[48] There is limited data on the readability and reliability of information about hypertension.[48] Studies have demonstrated that information on hypertension is of moderate reliability; further, the higher its reliability, the lower its readability.[49,50] Readability is critical for health information given the potential cognitive decline associated with aging.[39] Approximately 50% of the online content related to hypertension exceeds the recommended readability level.[49,50]

Older adults may have sensory issues such as visual and hearing impairment that may impact their communication skills.[17] Communication gaps with older adult patients can lead to feelings of disenfranchisement. Clinicians may be unaware of how aging impacts speaking and listening and can lead to patient feelings of isolation and neglect due to comprehension failure.[51] While this refers to verbal communication, it is one area that can be aided by digital health as information can be provided in a variety of written or verbal formats. When individuals are overreliant on stereotypes of older individuals, they may engage in "elderspeak," by deliberately using slow speech cadence, a higher pitched voice, and language that is often perceived as condescending.[52]

Table 1
Key stakeholders and their roles in public health messaging for hypertension

Stakeholders	Role
Individuals	1. Control blood pressure 2. Be physically active and try to do at least 150 min of moderately paced exercise weekly; eat healthy
Federal government	1. Research and implement innovative interventions 2. Create and fund policies that make hypertension control a priority 3. Expand public health insurance and employee plans to cover effective interventions 4. Increase access to healthy food and beverage options 5. Promote policies that lead to increased spaces for physical activity
State and local governments	1. Fund activities that address social determinants of health 2. Expand the scope of practice for nurses, pharmacists, and community health workers 3. Expand public health insurance and employee plans to cover effective interventions: cover home blood pressure monitors, reduce copays 4. Increase access to healthy food and beverage options 5. Enhance access to public spaces for walking 6. Promote policies that lead to increased spaces for physical activity 7. Support community programs that promote safe environments
Public health professionals	1. Convene quality improvement collaboratives that help clinical teams/systems achieve hypertension control 2. Work with public health insurance and employee plans to cover effective interventions 3. Conduct public health surveillance to identify high risk groups for uncontrolled hypertension 4. Invest in programs that link clinical services with community resources 5. Help individuals make lifestyle changes and obtain access to healthy food assistance 6. Promote policies that increase physical activity
Health care professionals	1. Implement protocols to standardize care 2. Refer all patients to lifestyle change resources 3. Teach self-measured blood pressure at home and follow-up about control 4. Simplify medication regimens and prescribe electronically to synchronize regimens 5. Use clinician dashboards to highlight gaps to be improved through quality improvement initiatives
Professional associations and societies	1. Develop national guidelines with targeted summaries for laypersons 2. Include guideline-based recommendations in training programs 3. Share guidelines and recommendations through continuing educational courses, publications, newsletters, and social media 4. Support and share policies that help improve blood pressure control

(continued on next page)

Table 1 *(continued)*	
Stakeholders	**Role**
Health care practices, health centers, and health systems	1. Ensure validated and calibrates automated blood pressure cuffs are present in all examination rooms 2. Provide regular training on the correct measurement of blood pressure 3. Implement protocols to standardize management 4. Use dashboards to highlight gaps to be improved through quality improvement initiatives and include hypertension control as a quality metric 5. Ensure all interventions are culturally and, linguistically appropriate and can be understood by those of any age with any degree of education
Health plans and managed care organizations	1. Reduce or eliminate out-of-pocket costs for antihypertensive medications 2. Provide coverage for automated home blood pressure kits 3. Reimburse providers for time spent teaching home blood pressure monitoring and following up on data submitted by patient logs 4. Reimburse pharmacists for time spent counseling about hypertension management 5. Expand access to prevention programs for patients 6. Provide incentives to clinicians and beneficiaries to encourage better blood pressure control
Employers and health plan purchasers	1. Select plans that reduce or eliminate out-of-pocket costs for antihypertensive medications 2. Select plans that provide coverage for automated home blood pressure kits 3. Provide support to employees to be more active at work or away from work 4. Provide healthy food and drink options 5. Provide virtual education for physical activity and nutrition
Academic institutions and researchers	1. Conduct effectiveness studies about hypertension management 2. Conduct research about the role of social determinants of health in hypertension 3. Develop programs in cardiovascular epidemiology and expand public health curricula to use data from electronic health records as a research tool 4. Increase research in implementation science, health systems, and policy assessment research to expand best practices
Community organizations, public-private partnerships, and foundations	1. Convene experts to develop guidelines 2. Support links between clinical services and community resources 3. Use organizational assets to address social determinants of health 4. Promote resources to support equity in blood pressure management 5. Support policies that make blood pressure management easier 6. Use multiple communication strategies to promote hypertension awareness and the importance of control

Adapted from: US Department of Health and Human Services. The Surgeon General's Call to Action to Control Hypertension. US Department of Health and Human Services, Office of the Surgeon General; 2020

While this should be avoided in verbal communication, technology may help in overcoming some of these issues including recorded messages that can be heard better by older adults and incorporate features that allow users to adjust speech rate and replay.[52]

POTENTIAL SOLUTIONS AND NOTABLE EXAMPLES OF EFFECTIVE STRATEGIES IN PUBLIC HEALTH MESSAGING

Many initiatives are directed toward encouraging patients to measure their BP. Many communities offer BP checks performed by emergency medical technicians or paramedics in fire stations and other locations. Additionally, many national retail chain pharmacies have services to perform BP checks.[51–66] Much of this information can be found on the Web sites of local health departments.

There are emerging data about how digital health tools can be used to remind patients to measure and record their BP. BP data can often be electronically shared with clinicians or summarized for health care visits. A number of remote monitoring programs have been shown to improve BP control.[53,54] For example, in the Brigham Protocol-Based Hypertension Optimization Program, 130 patients with hypertension were enrolled in a home-based BP control program executed by nonphysicians. Using remote BP monitoring and medication titration via telephone, 81% of all enrolled patients and 91% of patients who regularly measured their BP achieved target BP levels.[53] Meta-analyses suggest that remote monitoring can lead to significant improvements in BP control.[45]

Increasingly, telehealth and mobile health care applications are being used to improve access to care and provide follow-up recommendations.[30,45] However, digital content must be tailored to the needs of older adults.

Many landmark, randomized BP trials excluded older adults. Clinical trials that included older adults are SPRINT (A Randomized Trial of Intensive versus Standard Blood Pressure-Control),[23] HYVET (Treatment of Hypertension in Patients 80 Years of Age or Older),[24] and SHEP (The Systolic Hypertension in the Elderly Program),[55] but participants were generally healthier and had fewer comorbidities.[22,56] To address these gaps, the US Food and Drug Administration has created a "Roadmap to 2030 for the Evaluation of New Drugs in Older Adults."[57] This roadmap emphasizes the need to minimize unnecessary exclusion criteria in clinical trials, eliminate obstacles to trial participation, and develop studies that specifically address the clinical outcomes and safety concerns of older patients. The success of this initiative will rely on the integration of various data sources, the reorganization of clinical trial support, and the provision of access to a diverse group of underrepresented individuals, including older adults.[57,58]

Future research should prioritize investigating the management of cardiovascular disease in the older population, including the development of suitable care models. Currently, there is a lack of evidence in this area, highlighting the need for further exploration. Part of this change should be driven by federal and state governments and insurance programs. Many older patients rely on fixed incomes and participate in insurance programs sponsored by both federal and state governments. This change in health care coverage might lead to a decrease in accessibility to certain treatments and services. Furthermore, elderly patients frequently transition into assisted living facilities or residential homes. These housing arrangements could create obstacles to receiving care, since getting to medical appointments at the clinic might be too expensive or challenging to coordinate. These difficulties could worsen therapeutic inertia or further marginalize elderly individuals.[39]

Clinician training is a widely employed approach to tackle these issues.[10,59] While continuing medical education initiatives are commonly utilized, there is insufficient proof of their effectiveness. Direct outreach visits by a knowledgeable individual to provide information and feedback on clinician performance can help decrease therapeutic inertia and prove to be economical.[10,29] It is essential for clinicians to educate patients on BP and rectify any misconceptions. Moreover, the dissemination of guidelines plays a crucial role in communication. There has been a concerted effort by the ACC and AHA to disseminate clinical guidelines, improve readability for clinicians and laypersons, and provide point-of-care access through smartphone applications.[29] Team-based care models incorporating physicians, advanced practice providers, nurses, and pharmacists are recommended and can improve access to care, risk factor control, and bridge the gaps in care to high-risk groups; community health workers and lay-persons can complement health care teams.[20,21,42,45,53]

Notable Examples

There exist numerous public health strategies to involve older adults in discussions regarding hypertension. The "Hypertension Communications Kit (https://www.cdc.gov/dhdsp/pubs/toolkits/hmp-toolkit/index.ht)"[27] developed by the Centers for Disease Control and Prevention (CDC) offers a range of social media messaging, graphics, and additional resources. These valuable tools can be utilized by both public and private health care organizations, as well as public health agencies, to enhance their messaging campaigns.

The New York City Department of Health and Mental Hygiene has developed a "Hypertension Coaching Guide"[60] which offers simple language and effective strategies for involving patients in discussions about their BP. This guide includes common questions, concerns, and feedback from patients, as well as suitable, patient-focused responses that clinicians can utilize.

The Million Hearts 2027[61] (https://millionhearts.hhs.gov) program is national collaborative effort between the CDC and the Centers for Medicare & Medicaid Services. The primary objective of this program is to prevent 1 million avoidable cardiovascular deaths from occurring between the years 2022 and 2026. One of the major initiatives is centered around BP and offers a range of tools and resources for clinicians, public health practitioners, and patients.

Similarly, Target: BP[62] (https://targetbp.org/) is a national initiative led by the AHA and American Medical Association (AMA). It offers an extensive array of educational materials and practical resources to seamlessly integrate self BP monitoring into clinical workflows, aiding health care professionals and organizations in accurately diagnosing and treating hypertension.

FUTURE DIRECTIONS AND RESEARCH NEEDS

From a clinician's perspective, optimizing hypertension management for older patients is hindered by high therapeutic inertia and lack of multidisciplinary geriatric care. Although there are various tools available to tackle therapeutic inertia, there is a lack of well-defined best practices, which necessitates further research. Furthermore, there is a need for wider dissemination of current practice guidelines and recommendations. Resolving these challenges will require not only improvements in public health messaging but also changes in public policy regarding coverage for services and the promotion of research focused on the care of older patients.[29,39]

Increasing health literacy is a significant challenge from the perspective of patients. The methods to assess and determine the level of health literacy are not clear and may vary depending on race/ethnicity and socioeconomic status. Patient education can greatly benefit from the use of plain language tools, and there are numerous high-quality informational resources available for both patients and clinicians. Many of these resources are developed by national organizations such as the CDC, AHA, and AMA. In today's digital age, the rapid dissemination of information online presents an opportunity to raise awareness about hypertension and facilitate patient-clinician communication. However, it is important to find better ways to promote accurate information online.

Several interventions have been created to tackle hypertension within the community and involve older patients. It is essential for future studies to evaluate their efficacy, cost-effectiveness, and scalability. The Surgeon General's "Call to Action to Control Hypertension"[44] offers a comprehensive summary of key stakeholders and potential future paths they can pursue (see **Table 1**). This endeavor requires collaboration among governmental agencies, clinicians, insurance companies, technology firms, and community health workers.

SUMMARY

The prevalence of hypertension is highest among the older population and will continue to increase. Public health messaging plays a vital role in raising awareness and providing education on hypertension. Although progress has been made, there are still considerable areas for improvement. These approaches should involve customizing messages to cater to different demographic groups, incorporating digital health resources, advocating for regular health examinations, and acknowledging the role of caregivers. By adopting a comprehensive and individualized approach, communication can be more impactful, enabling older adults to effectively manage hypertension and enhance their overall health and wellness.

CLINICS CARE POINTS

- Hypertension in older adults should be treated per local guidelines. In the United States, per ACC/AHA guidelines, this is a goal systolic BP less than 130 mm Hg in those greater than 65 year old.

- Frailty should be assessed as part of shared decision-making when treating older adults for hypertension. The 2023 ESH guidelines offer a framework for assessing frailty and how that should frame hypertension treatment.

- Public health messaging to older adults should consider sensory and cognitive changes that may occur with aging. Individual providers should remain cognizant of this too when talking to patients.

- Community resources such as fire departments and pharmacies often can help screen for hypertension. Utilizing community resources such as places of worship can help educate individuals about hypertension and the need for treatment. These resources should be incorporated into public health campaigns.

- The digital era provides opportunity for providers to engage in ongoing medical education. It also is a frequent source of information for patients. To that end, digital information that is accurate and at an appropriate comprehension level should be prioritized. The best source for this information is national organizations such as the AHA.

DISCLOSURE

Dr J.A. Spitz has no disclosures. Dr E. Yang reports a relationship with the ACC, Genentech, Mineralys, Qure.ai, and Sky Labs that includes consulting/honoraria. Dr E.

Yang reports a relationship with Microsoft, United States that includes research grants. Dr E. Yang reports a relationship with Clocktree, Measure Labs, and TenPoint7 that includes consulting or advisory and equity or stocks. Dr R.S. Blumenthal has no disclosures. Dr G. Sharma is supported by AHA979472.

REFERENCES

1. Virani SS, Alonso A, Aparicio HJ, et al. Heart disease and stroke statistics—2021 update. Circulation 2021;143(8). https://doi.org/10.1161/cir.0000000000000950.
2. Whelton PK, Fuchs FD. High blood pressure and cardiovascular disease. Hypertension 2020. https://doi.org/10.1161/HYPERTENSIONAHA.119.14240.
3. Stamler J, Stamler R, Neaton JD. Blood pressure, systolic and Diastolic, and cardiovascular risks: US population data. Arch Intern Med 1993;153(5):598–615.
4. Verdecchia P, Angeli F, Reboldi G. Atrial fibrillation coronary artery disease hypertension myocardial infarction stroke Hypertension and Atrial Fibrillation Doubts and Certainties from Basic and Clinical Studies. Circ Res 2024. https://doi.org/10.1161/CIRCRESAHA.117.311402.
5. He J, Whelton PK. Elevated systolic blood pressure and risk of cardiovascular and renal disease: overview of evidence from observational epidemiologic studies and randomized controlled trials. Am Heart J 1999;138(3 Pt 2):211–9.
6. Abdi S, Spann A, Borilovic J, et al. Understanding the care and support needs of older people: a scoping review and categorisation using the WHO international classification of functioning, disability and health framework (ICF). BMC Geriatr 2019;19(1). https://doi.org/10.1186/s12877-019-1189-9.
7. Jaeger BC, Chen L, Foti K, et al. Hypertension statistics for US adults: an Opensource Web application for analysis and Visualization of national health and Nutrition examination survey data. Hypertension 2023;80(6):1311.
8. Richter D, Guasti L, Walker D, et al. Frailty in cardiology: definition, assessment and clinical implications for general cardiology. A consensus document of the Council for Cardiology practice (CCP), association for Acute Cardio Vascular care (ACVC), association of cardiovascular nursing and Allied Professions (AC-NAP), European association of preventive Cardiology (EAPC), European heart Rhythm association (EHRA), Council on Valvular heart diseases (VHD), Council on hypertension (CHT), Council of Cardio-Oncology (CCO), working group (WG) Aorta and Peripheral Vascular diseases, WG e-Cardiology, WG Thrombosis, of the European society of Cardiology, European primary care Cardiology society (EPCCS). Eur J Prev Cardiol 2020;29(1):216.
9. Guasti L, Ambrosetti M, Ferrari M, et al. Management of hypertension in the elderly and Frail patient. Drugs Aging 2022;39(10):763.
10. Dixon DL, Sharma G, Sandesara PB, et al. Therapeutic inertia in cardiovascular disease prevention. J Am Coll Cardiol 2019;74(13):1728.
11. Pollack Porter KM, Rutkow L, Mcginty EE. The importance of policy change for addressing public health Problems. Public Health Rep 2018;133(1_suppl):9S.
12. Pink SL, Stagnaro MN, Chu J, et al. The effects of short messages encouraging prevention behaviors early in the COVID-19 pandemic. PLoS One 2023;18(4).
13. Redwood H. Hypertension, society, and public policy 2007;9(suppl_B):B13.
14. Gifford JrR. Managing hypertension in the elderly: dispelling the myths. Cleve Clin J Med 1995;62:29–35.
15. Chirico F, Teixeira Da Silva JA. Evidence-based policies in public health to address COVID-19 vaccine hesitancy. Future Virol 2023;18(4):261.

16. Morrison FP, Kukafka R, Johnson SB. Analyzing the structure and content of public health messages. AMIA Annu Symp Proc 2005;2005:540–4.

17. Institute of Medicine. Communicating to advance the Public's health: Workshop summary. Washington, DC: The National Academies Press; 2015.

18. Martin SS, Aday AW, Almarzooq ZI, et al. On behalf of the American heart association Council on Epidemioloqy and prevention Sta-tistics Committee and stroke Statistics Subcommittee. 2024 heart disease and stroke statistics: a report of US and global data from the American heart association. Circulation 2024. https://doi.org/10.1161/CIR.0000000000001209.

19. Okonofua EC, Simpson KN, Jesri A, et al. Therapeutic inertia is an Impediment to achieving the healthy people 2010 blood pressure control goals. Hypertension 2006;47(3):345.

20. Whelton PK, Carey RM, Aronow WS, et al. 2017 ACC/AHA/AAPA/ABC/ACPM/AGS/APhA/ASH/ASPC/NMA/PCNA guideline for the prevention, detection, evaluation, and management of high blood pressure in adults: a report of the American College of cardiology/American heart association Task Force on clinical practice guidelines. Hypertension 2018;71(6):13.

21. Mancia G, Kreutz R, Brunström M, et al. 2023 ESH guidelines for the management of arterial hypertension the Task Force for the management of arterial hypertension of the European society of hypertension: Endorsed by the international society of hypertension (ISH) and the European renal association (ERA). J Hypertens 2023;41(12):1874–2071.

22. Oliveros E, Patel H, Kyung S, et al. Hypertension in older adults: assessment, management, and challenges. Clin Cardiol 2019;43(2):99.

23. Wright JT, Williamson JD, Whelton PK, et al. A randomized trial of intensive versus Standard blood-pressure control. N Engl J Med 2015;373(22):2103.

24. Beckett NS, Peters R, Fletcher AE, et al. Treatment of hypertension in patients 80 Years of age or older. N Engl J Med 2008. https://doi.org/10.1056/NEJMoa0801369.

25. Aïdoud A, Gana W, Poitau F, et al. High prevalence of geriatric conditions among older adults with cardiovascular disease. JAHA 2024;12(2). https://doi.org/10.1161/jaha.122.026850.

26. Benetos A, Petrovic M, Strandberg T. Compendium on the Pathophysiology and treatment of hypertension. Circ Res 2024. https://doi.org/10.1161/CIRCRESAHA.118.313236.

27. Hypertension management program (HMP) Toolkit, Available at: https://www.cdc.gov/dhdsp/pubs/toolkits/hmp-toolkit/index.htm. Accessed February 14, 2024.

28. Bryant KB, Sheppard JP, Ruiz-negrón N, et al. Impact of self-monitoring of blood pressure on Processes of hypertension care and long-term blood pressure control. JAHA 2024;9(15). https://doi.org/10.1161/jaha.120.016174.

29. Chan WV, Pearson TA, Bennett GC, et al. ACC/AHA special report: clinical practice guideline implementation strategies: a summary of systematic reviews by the NHLBI Implementation Science Work Group: a report of the American College of Cardiology/American Heart Association Task Force on Clinical Practice Guidelines. Circulation 2017;135(9):e122-e137.

30. Guasti L, Dilaveris P, Mamas MA, et al. Digital health in older adults for the prevention and management of cardiovascular diseases and frailty. A clinical consensus statement from the ESC Council for Cardiology Practice/Taskforce on Geriatric Cardiology, the ESC Digital Health Committee and the ESC Working Group on e-Cardiology. ESC Heart Failure 2022;9(5):2808.

31. Rochat L, Wilkosc-Debczynska M, Zajac-Lamparska L, et al. Internet Use and Problematic Use in Seniors: a Comparative study in Switzerland and Poland. Front. Psychiatry. 2021;12. https://doi.org/10.3389/fpsyt.2021.609190.

32. Onyeaka HK, Romero P, Healy BC, et al. Age Differences in the Use of health information technology among adults in the United States: an analysis of the health information national trends survey. J Aging Health 2020;33(1–2):147.

33. Han M, Tan XY, Lee R, et al. Impact of social media on health-related outcomes among older adults in Singapore: Qualitative study. JMIR Aging. 2021;4(1). https://doi.org/10.2196/23826.

34. Turner AM, Osterhage KP, Taylor JO, et al. A Closer Look at Health Information Seeking by Older Adults and Involved Family and Friends: Design Considerations for Health Information Technologies. AMIA Annu Symp Proc 2018;2018: 1036–45.

35. Office of Disease Prevention and Health Promotion. U.S. Department of Health and Human Services, Social determinants of health and older adults. health.gov Web site, Available at: https://health.gov/our-work/national-health-initiatives/healthy-aging/social-determinants-health-and-older-adults#:~:text=Social%20determinants%20of%20health%20(SDOH,of%2Dlife%20outcomes%20and%20risks. Accessed February 14, 2024.

36. Akinyelure OP, Jaeger BC, Oparil S, et al. Social determinants of health and Uncontrolled blood pressure in a national cohort of Black and white US adults: the REGARDS study. Hypertension 2023;80(7):1403.

37. Perez FP, Perez CA, Chumbiauca MN. Insights into the social determinants of health in older adults. JBiSE 2022;15(11):261.

38. Lester PE, Dharmarajan TS, Weinstein E. The Looming geriatrician Shortage: Ramifications and solutions. J Aging Health 2019;32(9):1052.

39. Goyal P, Kwak MJ, Al Malouf C, et al. Geriatric cardiology: Coming of age. JACC (J Am Coll Cardiol): Advances 2022;1(3).

40. Health Resources and Services Administration. Health Workforce Projections.

41. Victor RG, Lynch K, Li N, et al. A Cluster-randomized trial of blood-pressure reduction in Black barbershops. N Engl J Med 2018;378(14):1291.

42. Schoenthaler AM, Lancaster KJ, Chaplin W, et al. Cluster randomized clinical trial of FAITH (Faith-Based approaches in the treatment of hypertension) in Blacks. Circ: Cardiovascular Quality and Outcomes 2024;11(10). https://doi.org/10.1161/circoutcomes.118.004691.

43. Chantakeeree C, Sormunen M, Jullamate P, et al. Understanding perspectives on health-promoting behaviours among older adults with hypertension. Int J Qual Stud Health Well-Being 2022;17(1). https://doi.org/10.1080/17482631.2022.2103943.

44. U.S. Department of Health and Human Services. The Surgeon General's Call to action to control hypertension. U.S. Department of Health and Human Services, Office of the Surgeon General; 2020.

45. Kario K. Management of hypertension in the digital era Small Wearable monitoring Devices for remote blood pressure monitoring. Hypertension 2020. https://doi.org/10.1161/HYPERTENSIONAHA.120.14742.

46. Centers for Disease Control and Prevention. Improving Health Literacy for Older Adults: Expert Panel Report 2009. 2009

47. Wändi Bruine dB, Okan Y, Krishnamurti T, et al. The role of confidence and knowledge in Intentions to (not) seek care for hypertension: evidence from a national survey. Med Decis Making 2023;43(4):461–77.

48. Silberg WM, Lundberg GD, Musacchio RA. Assessing, Controlling, and Assuring the Quality of Medical Information on the Internet: Caveant Lector et Viewor—Let the Reader and Viewer Beware. JAMA 1997;277(15):1244–5.
49. Tahir M, Usman M, Muhammad F, et al. Evaluation of quality and readability of on-line health information on high blood pressure using DISCERN and Flesch-Kincaid tools. Appl Sci 2020;10(9). https://doi.org/10.3390/app10093214.
50. Oloidi A, Nduaguba SO, Obamiro K. Assessment of quality and readability of internet-based health information related to commonly prescribed angiotensin receptor blockers. Pan Afr Med J 2020;35. https://doi.org/10.11604/pamj.2020.35.70.18237.
51. Ryan EB, Giles H, Bartolucci G, et al. Psycholinguistic and social psychological components of communication by and with the elderly. Lang Commun 1986; 6(1):1–24.
52. Kemper S, Lacal JC. Addressing the communication needs of an aging society. In: Pew RW, Van Hemel SB, editors. Technology for Adaptive aging. Washington, DC: National Academies Press (US); 2004.
53. Fisher NDL, Fera LE, Dunning JR, et al. Development of an entirely remote, non-physician led hypertension management program. Clin Cardiol 2019;42(2):285.
54. Clark D, Woods J, Zhang Y, et al. Home blood pressure Telemonitoring with remote hypertension management in a Rural and Low-income population. Hypertension 2021;78(6):1927.
55. Perry HM Jr, Davis BR, Price TR, et al. Effect of treating isolated systolic hypertension on the risk of developing various types and subtypes of stroke: the Systolic Hypertension in the Elderly Program (SHEP). JAMA 2000;284(4):465–71.
56. Rich MW, Chyun DA, Skolnick AH, et al. Knowledge gaps in cardiovascular care of the older adult population. Circulation 2024;133(21):2103.
57. Liu Q, Schwartz JB, Slattum PW, et al. Roadmap to 2030 for Drug evaluation in older adults. Clin Pharma and Therapeutics 2021;112(2):210.
58. Califf RM. Now is the time to fix the evidence generation system. Clin Trials 2023; 20(1):3.
59. Haff N, Sreedhara SK, Wood W, et al. Testing interventions to reduce clinical inertia in the treatment of hypertension: rationale and design of a pragmatic randomized controlled trial. Am Heart J 2024;268:18.
60. NYC Health, Effective communication strategies to manage hypertension: a hypertension Coaching guide, Available at: https://www.nyc.gov/assets/doh/downloads/pdf/csi/hyperkit-coaching-guide.pdf. Accessed February 14, 2024.
61. Million hearts, Available at: https://millionhearts.hhs.gov. Accessed February 14, 2024.
62. Target: BP, Available at: https://targetbp.org. Accessed February 14, 2024.
63. Office of Disease Prevention and Health Promotion. U.S. Department of Health and Human Services. Get Your blood pressure checked. Available at: health. gov https://health.gov/myhealthfinder/doctor-visits/screening-tests/get-your-blood-pressure-checked. Accessed February 14, 2024.
64. Dixon DL, Johnston K, Patterson J, et al. Cost-effectiveness of pharmacist Prescribing for managing hypertension in the United States. JAMA Netw Open 2023;6(11).
65. Blood pressure screening & Counseling. Walgreens, Available at: https://www.walgreens.com/topic/pharmacy/scheduler/blood-pressure-screening-and-counseling_8.jsp. Accessed February 14, 2024.
66. High blood pressure screening. CVS, Available at: https://www.cvs.com/minuteclinic/services/high-blood-pressure-evaluation. Accessed February 14, 2024.

UNITED STATES POSTAL SERVICE®

Statement of Ownership, Management, and Circulation (All Periodicals Publications Except Requester Publications)

1. Publication Title	2. Publication Number	3. Filing Date
CLINICS IN GERIATRIC MEDICINE	000 – 704	9/18/2024

4. Issue Frequency	5. Number of Issues Published Annually	6. Annual Subscription Price
FEB, MAY, AUG, NOV	4	$321.00

7. Complete Mailing Address of Known Office of Publication (Not printer) (Street, city, county, state, and ZIP+4®)

ELSEVIER INC.
230 Park Avenue, Suite 800
New York, NY 10169

Contact Person
Malathi Samayan

Telephone (Include area code)
91-44-4299-4507

8. Complete Mailing Address of Headquarters or General Business Office of Publisher (Not printer)

ELSEVIER INC.
230 Park Avenue, Suite 800
New York, NY 10169

9. Full Names and Complete Mailing Addresses of Publisher, Editor, and Managing Editor (Do not leave blank)

Publisher (Name and complete mailing address)

Dolores Meloni, ELSEVIER INC.
1600 JOHN F KENNEDY BLVD. SUITE 1600
PHILADELPHIA, PA 19103-2899

Editor (Name and complete mailing address)

Taylor Hayes, ELSEVIER INC.
1600 JOHN F KENNEDY BLVD. SUITE 1600
PHILADELPHIA, PA 19103-2899

Managing Editor (Name and complete mailing address)

PATRICK MANLEY, ELSEVIER INC.
1600 JOHN F KENNEDY BLVD. SUITE 1600
PHILADELPHIA, PA 19103-2899

10. Owner (Do not leave blank. If the publication is owned by a corporation, give the name and address of the corporation immediately followed by the names and addresses of all stockholders owning or holding 1 percent or more of the total amount of stock. If not owned by a corporation, give the names and addresses of the individual owners. If owned by a partnership or other unincorporated firm, give its name and address as well as those of each individual owner. If the publication is published by a nonprofit organization, give its name and address.)

Full Name	Complete Mailing Address
WHOLLY OWNED SUBSIDIARY OF REED/ELSEVIER, US HOLDINGS	1600 JOHN F KENNEDY BLVD. SUITE 1600 PHILADELPHIA, PA 19103-2899

11. Known Bondholders, Mortgagees, and Other Security Holders Owning or Holding 1 Percent or More of Total Amount of Bonds, Mortgages, or Other Securities. If none, check box ▸ ☐ None

Full Name	Complete Mailing Address
N/A	

12. Tax Status (For completion by nonprofit organizations authorized to mail at nonprofit rates) (Check one)
The purpose, function, and nonprofit status of this organization and the exempt status for federal income tax purposes:

☒ Has Not Changed During Preceding 12 Months
☐ Has Changed During Preceding 12 Months (Publisher must submit explanation of change with this statement)

PS Form 3526, July 2014 (Page 1 of 4 (see instructions page 4)) PSN: 7530-01-000-9931 PRIVACY NOTICE: See our privacy policy on www.usps.com.

13. Publication Title	14. Issue Date for Circulation Data Below
CLINICS IN GERIATRIC MEDICINE	AUGUST 2024

15. Extent and Nature of Circulation			Average No. Copies Each Issue During Preceding 12 Months	No. Copies of Single Issue Published Nearest to Filing Date
a. Total Number of Copies (Net press run)			79	67
b. Paid Circulation (By Mail and Outside the Mail)	(1)	Mailed Outside-County Paid Subscriptions Stated on PS Form 3541 (Include paid distribution above nominal rate, advertiser's proof copies, and exchange copies)	47	36
	(2)	Mailed In-County Paid Subscriptions Stated on PS Form 3541 (Include paid distribution above nominal rate, advertiser's proof copies, and exchange copies)	0	0
	(3)	Paid Distribution Outside the Mails Including Sales Through Dealers and Carriers, Street Vendors, Counter Sales, and Other Paid Distribution Outside USPS®	23	24
	(4)	Paid Distribution by Other Classes of Mail Through the USPS (e.g. First-Class Mail®)	8	6
c. Total Paid Distribution (Sum of 15b (1), (2), (3), and (4))			78	66
d. Free or Nominal Rate Distribution (By Mail and Outside the Mail)	(1)	Free or Nominal Rate Outside-County Copies included on PS Form 3541	0	0
	(2)	Free or Nominal Rate In-County Copies Included on PS Form 3541	0	0
	(3)	Free or Nominal Rate Copies Mailed at Other Classes Through the USPS (e.g. First-Class Mail)	0	0
	(4)	Free or Nominal Rate Distribution Outside the Mail (Carriers or other means)	1	1
e. Total Free or Nominal Rate Distribution (Sum of 15d (1), (2), (3) and (4))			1	1
f. Total Distribution (Sum of 15c and 15e)			79	67
g. Copies not Distributed (See Instructions to Publishers #4 (page #3))			0	0
h. Total (Sum of 15f and g)			79	67
i. Percent Paid (15c divided by 15f times 100)			98.73%	98.51%

* If you are claiming electronic copies, go to line 16 on page 3. If you are not claiming electronic copies, skip to line 17 on page 3.

PS Form 3526, July 2014 (Page 2 of 4)

16. Electronic Copy Circulation	Average No. Copies Each Issue During Preceding 12 Months	No. Copies of Single Issue Published Nearest to Filing Date
a. Paid Electronic Copies ▸		
b. Total Paid Print Copies (Line 15c) + Paid Electronic Copies (Line 16a) ▸		
c. Total Print Distribution (Line 15f) + Paid Electronic Copies (Line 16a) ▸		
d. Percent Paid (Both Print & Electronic Copies) (16b divided by 16c × 100) ▸		

☒ I certify that 50% of all my distributed copies (electronic and print) are paid above a nominal price.

17. Publication of Statement of Ownership

☒ If the publication is a general publication, publication of this statement is required. Will be printed in the NOVEMBER 2024 issue of this publication. ☐ Publication not required.

18. Signature and Title of Editor, Publisher, Business Manager, or Owner		Date
Malathi Samayan - Distribution Controller	*Malathi Samayan*	9/18/2024

I certify that all information furnished on this form is true and complete. I understand that anyone who furnishes false or misleading information on this form or who omits material or information requested on the form may be subject to criminal sanctions (including fines and imprisonment) and/or civil sanctions (including civil penalties).

PS Form 3526, July 2014 (Page 3 of 4) PRIVACY NOTICE: See our privacy policy on www.usps.com

Moving?

Make sure your subscription moves with you!

To notify us of your new address, find your **Clinics Account Number** (located on your mailing label above your name), and contact customer service at:

Email: journalscustomerservice-usa@elsevier.com

800-654-2452 (subscribers in the U.S. & Canada)
314-447-8871 (subscribers outside of the U.S. & Canada)

Fax number: 314-447-8029

Elsevier Health Sciences Division
Subscription Customer Service
3251 Riverport Lane
Maryland Heights, MO 63043

*To ensure uninterrupted delivery of your subscription, please notify us at least 4 weeks in advance of move.

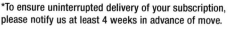

Printed and bound by CPI Group (UK) Ltd, Croydon, CR0 4YY

08/05/2025

01864752-0008